Introduction to
Symbolic and Augmentative
Communication

Introduction to Symbolic and Augmentative Communication

Stephen von Tetzchner
and Harald Martinsen
University of Oslo, Norway

Translated by Kevin M.J. Quirk

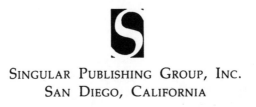

SINGULAR PUBLISHING GROUP, INC.
SAN DIEGO, CALIFORNIA

© 1992 Whurr Publishers
First published, in English, 1992 by
Whurr Publishers Ltd
19b Compton Terrace, London N1 2UN, England
First published in Norwegian, 1991, by Gyldendal, Oslo, Norway
Published and distributed in the United States and Canada by
SINGULAR PUBLISHING GROUP, INC.
4284 41st Street
San Diego, California 92105, USA
Reprinted 1993

Adult performing manual signs drawn by Kristin Torp
Other manual signs drawn by Astyrid H. Støren
Other drawings by Tom Nordli

Library of Congress Cataloging in Publication Data
Tetzchner. Stephen von.
    Introduction to symbolic and augmentative communication /
by Stephen von Tetzchner and Harald Martinsen.
        p. cm.
    Includes bibliographical references and index.
    ISBN 1-56593-050-9
    1. Communication devices for the disabled. 2. Visual
communication. 3. Sign language. 4. Language disorders.
5. Disabled--Means of communication. I. Martinsen. Harald.
II. Title
RC429. T48 1992
616. 85' 503--dc20

Photoset by Stephen Cary
Printed and bound in the UK by
Athenaeum Press Ltd, Newcastle upon Tyne

Preface

Manual and graphic signs are now in common use among hearing people who have severe developmental speech and language difficulties. Hence, an increasing number of professionals and family members are involved with children, adolescents and adults who use such communication forms, and they need to know about alternative communication systems and their use.

In the Nordic countries, a need was expressed for an introductory textbook comprising a breakdown of the needs of different user groups and, in addition, a variety of communication systems and instructional methods. One of the purposes of this book is to facilitate collaboration between different professionals, and between families and professionals. It may serve as an introductory textbook for speech and language therapists, teachers, psychologists, care nurses, etc, as well as for families of people with speech and language disabilities.

For both professionals and family members, it is important to have access to professional books in their own language. The present volume was first written in Norwegian to provide a textbook for the Norwegian-, Danish- and Swedish-speaking audiences. However, British and North American colleagues informed us that there was a need for this kind of introductory textbook in their countries, and encouraged us to translate it into English.

The present volume has been adapted to the English-speaking communities. The illustrations of manual signs are drawings of British Sign Language. We are thankful to Mike Martin of The Royal National Institute for Deaf People for providing us with sign dictionaries and helping us with signs not included in the dictionaries. Pictogram symbols have proved very useful in the Nordic countries, and we want to thank Subhas Maharaj for his kind permission to use a large number of them to illustrate this book. For technical reasons, the Pictogram symbols in this volume are based on the Norwegian version, a few of these being slightly different from the Canadian originals.

Stephen von Tetzchner
Harald Martinsen

Contents

Chapter 1
Introduction

A significant portion of the population is unable to communicate with the aid of speech. Among those afflicted are children, adolescents and adults with motor disabilities, mental handicap, autism, delayed speech and other developmental or acquired language disorders. The size of this group is not fully known. Those with acquired impairments constitute an extensive group, including many elderly people. The present book is mainly concerned with developmental language and communication disorders. This sub-group may be estimated to include at least 0.5 per cent of the population, although this estimate is probably low. In the last two decades there has been more focus on language and communication disorders, and the number of cases has subsequently increased.

People who are unable to communicate with the aid of speech share the need for an alternative communication system. The growing interest in language and communication disorders has also led to an increased awareness of the need for such systems. Today there are a large number of systems available.

Among other issues, this book is concerned with the use of manual signs in language intervention. The largest group of people who use signs are those who are deaf. Deaf children, however, acquire sign language in the same informal manner as most hearing children learn to speak. Growing up in a signing environment, they do not need any special teaching to learn to sign. Consequently, the present book is *not* concerned with deaf people.

There are great differences among those in need of an alternative communication system. Many children will develop speech, and their need for alternative systems will disappear. To various degrees, they also adapt to society and become ordinary members of a social community.

For children with a lifelong need for an alternative communication system, language comprehension and motor skills may determine their course of life and the degree to which they will attain a normal quality of life.

A large sub-group understands fully what other people say and the ongoing events that affect them, and shares the values and norms of the prevailing culture. Their need for an alternative communication system is due to motor impairments that hinder speech. Usually, they have motor disorders that hinder other activities as well, making them dependent on technical aids and help from other people.

Those who fail to acquire speech and do not profit from traditional speech therapy need an alternative communication system too. For most of the people in this group, the language disorder is part of a more general impairment that also influences other intellectual and social skills.

Difficulty in communicating with other people produces widespread consequences and affects people in all walks of life and at all ages. In the pre-lingual period, communication difficulties influence the interaction between the children and their caregivers, and disturb or destroy natural socialisation processes. Parents of children with extensive communication disorders often experience a lack of contact with their children. They have problems understanding their children's interests and are often confused. The children risk losing opportunities for natural learning which normally form part of any social environment. Most of what children learn as they grow up is transmitted through reactions from adults and other children, what others explain and tell them about things, and what others say and do. In this manner, children learn language and acquire the knowledge, values and norms of their culture. Children with language and communication disorders have less exposure than others to such learning opportunities.

From childhood and throughout life, feelings of self-sufficiency, self-respect and worth are closely related to the ability to express oneself. The perception of oneself as independent and equal to others is related to the ability to tell of one's needs, concerns and feelings. People who are unable to do this lose control over their own fate. Their experience is that other people underestimate them – talk down to them, humour them, and make decisions for them – thus reinforcing their feeling of being second-class citizens. For the most severely disabled, such negative experiences may – together with inconsistent and infrequent reactions to their wants – lead to learned passivity and extensive dependency on others. For them, the ability to communicate means an increased understanding of the world, the possibility of expressing their needs, and a higher level of activity. Providing an alternative mode of communication for speechless children and adults increases their quality of life.

People with extensive motor impairments often learn communication more rapidly than other skills. For them, the language skills they acquire may have a dual function, enabling them to participate more in a broad range of activities that are not usually dependent on such skills.

The choice of an alternative communication system must be viewed in a broad perspective. The system should improve everyday life and make the user feel less handicapped and more able to master life. The choice of communication system must therefore be based on the total needs of the individual. Most people who need an alternative communication system also need other forms of intervention. The teaching of a new communication system must also be coordinated with the whole range of services on offer, such as education, training and help, etc. Language and communication intervention must not be isolated from other forms of intervention. Just as with other forms of language and communication, the alternative communication system should function as a tool to be used in all life situations.

Many new communication systems and aids have come into use, and it has been difficult to find descriptions and evaluations of them. Since the various groups of people in need of alternative communication often require different communication systems, knowledge of what systems are available is crucial in order to be able to make the right decisions. It is also necessary to know how to adapt the different systems and aids to the needs of individual users. Thus, the main aims of this book are to:

give an overview of communication systems and communication aids that can be used with children, adolescents and adults in need of alternative forms of communication

give an overview of the principal groups of people in need of an alternative communication form, and the major differences between individuals within the various groups

describe factors that are important for the choice of communication system and individual signs, and discuss how the choice can be based as much as possible on the user's particular characteristics and needs

describe the most important principles for teaching the different alternative communication systems. This also includes a discussion of how language and communication intervention may best be adapted to enhance the initiative and self-reliance of the individual.

Terminology and notation

In written presentations of sign language, every sign has a *gloss*, i.e. a name or translation. Such glosses are usually written in capital letters: for example, SHOP. Some signs need more than one word in translation, and when the gloss for a single sign contains two or more words, these are hyphenated: for example, YOU-AND-ME. This notation is used for both manual and graphic signs. Spoken words, as well as words that are spelled or written with ordinary letters, are italicised, for example, *H-e-l-l-o* or *Hello*. The meaning of a word, sign or sentence is set in quotation marks. For example, YOU-AND-ME SHOP may mean 'You and I are going shopping'.

Figure 1. *Notation in use in this book. WE-TWO SHOP, or YOU I SHOP, may mean 'We are going shopping'.*

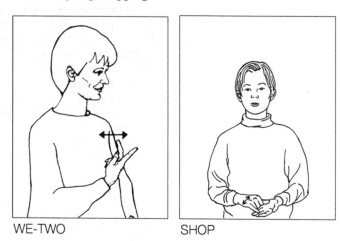

WE-TWO   SHOP

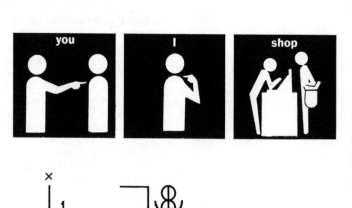

we, us   shop

Although most of the users are children, many adolescents are also taught to use alternative communication. One reason for this is that many people with severe disabilities need intervention into adulthood – and some throughout their life. Another reason is that there is still a substantial group of adults who never had the opportunity to learn an alternative communication system in childhood. We therefore use the term *individual* to refer to the person who receives intervention, unless it is clear from the context that it is a child, an adolescent or an adult. We use the term *teacher* for any professional involved in teaching the individual. Thus, a 'teacher' may be a nursery school teacher, teacher, care nurse, speech therapist, psychologist, etc.

Chapter 2
Augmentative and alternative communication

The use of graphic and manual signs by non-deaf people with language and communication disorders is fairly new, and there is therefore a need for new terms. In order to simplify communication in this area, there is a move towards the standardisation of terminology (see Bloomberg and Lloyd, 1986). The words and expressions used in this book mainly follow the international standard.

In keeping with international terminology, phrases such as 'to speak', 'to say something', 'speaker' and 'listener', etc., are used fairly loosely. An 'aided speaker' uses a communication aid, while a 'natural speaker' speaks in the normal manner. A 'listener' is the same as a partner in a conversation. A 'listener' does not necessarily hear somebody speak, but may be written to or communicated with in some other way.

The term 'sign' is the generic term for linguistic forms that are not speech, and includes both manual signs and graphic signs.

> *Manual signs* include sign language for deaf people and other signs performed with the hands (for example, Signed Norwegian and Seeing Exact English). *Sign language* comprises only manual signs, while *sign systems* may be used to describe both manual signs and graphic signs.

> *Graphic signs* include all graphically formed signs (Blissymbols, PIC signs, etc.). Signs that are made of wood or plastic (Premack's word bricks) are also regarded as graphic signs.

In the literature on augmentative communication, graphic signs have often been described as 'symbols'. In the field of linguistics, however, both speech and manual and graphic signs are referred to as language symbols. Using the word 'symbol' to describe only one of these groups is therefore imprudent. It is also worth noting that Pierce (1931), among others, distinguishes between 'symbolic' and 'iconic' signs. The majority of the graphic signs described as 'symbol systems' would not be regarded as 'symbolic' by

Pierce. The symbol concept is thus both unclear and disputed, and 'sign' would seem to be a more neutral concept (cf. Remington and Light, 1983).

Alternative communication is used when the individual communicates in face-to-face communication in other ways than through speech. Manual and graphic signs, Morse code, writing, etc., are alternative forms of communication for individuals who lack the ability to speak.

Speech is the best and most common form of communication for people with normal hearing. However, not everyone is able to speak, no matter how much training they are given. For these individuals, alternative communication will be their main form of communication. Others have more limited speech disorders. They may need alternative communication while learning to speak or in order to make their speech easier to understand.

Augmentative communication means supplementary or supportive communication. The word augmentative emphasises the fact that training in alternative forms of communication has a dual purpose: to promote and supplement speech and to guarantee an alternative form of communication if the individual does not begin to speak.

The division between aided and unaided, and between dependent and independent communication, designates different forms of augmentative communication.

Aided communication includes all forms of communication in which the linguistic expression exists in a physical form external to the user. The signs are *selected*. Pointing boards, synthetic speech machines, computers and other forms of communication aids all belong to this category. Pointing at a graphic sign or picture is a form of aided communication because the sign or picture is the communicative expression.

Unaided communication is communication in which the individual communicating must make the linguistic expressions without such help. The signs are *produced*. This chiefly encompasses manual signs, but Morse code also belongs to this category because the user himself makes every single letter in Morse. Blinking with one's eyes to indicate 'yes' and 'no' is also a form of unaided communication. The same applies to pointing at an object, for example, because the pointing is the communicative expression.

Dependent communication means that the individual communicating relies on another person to put together or interpret what is being said. This may occur with the help of boards depicting single letters, words or graphic signs.

Independent communication means that the message is wholly formulated by the user. This may be done with the help of synthetic speech machines that speak whole sentences, or technical aids where the communicated message is written on paper or a screen.

Manual signs

Most countries have two main types of manual signs. The first type is found in the sign languages used among deaf people. These sign languages are often named after the country: for example, Norwegian sign language (NSL) and American sign language (ASL). Sign languages have their own grammar, with inflections and word orders (syntax) that differ from that of spoken languages. The sign languages of the various countries differ in much the same way as the spoken languages do. The topography (articulation) of the signs differs, they are inflected differently and the sentences have a different word order. There are also dialectal variations. Sign languages have developed naturally and have undergone change through contact with other sign languages, as well as with spoken and written languages (cf. Klima and Bellugi, 1979; Martinsen, Nordeng and von Tetzchner, 1985).

The other type of sign language is constructed to follow speech word for word. They are also inflected in the same way as the spoken language (cf. Wilbur, 1979). These sign languages – signed Norwegian, signed English, etc. – are often devised by teachers of the deaf as a means of representing the spoken language with the aid of signs. Usually, many of the signs in the constructed sign languages are borrowed from sign languages for deaf people, while inflections and syntax are modelled upon the national spoken language. This type of sign language has never been used widely among deaf people because the inflections and syntax are not well suited to a visual and manual language.

In the training of non-deaf individuals with a communicative disability, the sign language that follows the spoken language is commonly used. This is done for several reasons: there are few non-deaf people who have a command of the sign language for deaf people, the majority of national sign languages are not described in sufficient detail, and there is a lack of suitable teaching material. This also applies to British sign language.

The ability to learn a new language varies, and many people find it a struggle. Learning a sign language that closely resembles speech is easier when one has a command of the spoken language. It is considerably more difficult to learn a language that has a totally different grammar. Using both signs and speech together will also be easier. For people with a good command of signing, a sign language that follows the spoken language will, however, be less effective in use than a natural sign language.

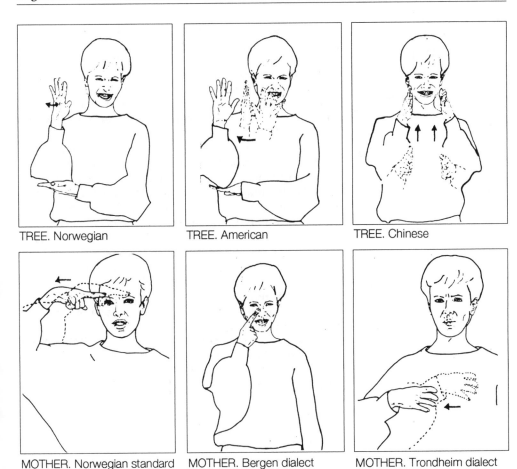

TREE. Norwegian   TREE. American   TREE. Chinese

MOTHER. Norwegian standard   MOTHER. Bergen dialect   MOTHER. Trondheim dialect

Graphic signs

Graphic sign systems are often linked to the use of communication aids ranging from simple pointing boards to apparatus based on advanced computer technology. Blissymbols and Premack's word bricks were two of the first systems to be used, but quite a number of systems have come into existence in the course of time (cf. Bloomberg and Lloyd, 1986). Only the most common of them will be dealt with here.

Blissymbols

Blissymbols are a form of *logographic* writing, i.e. written signs that are not based on a combination of letters. This means that the word, not the letter, becomes the smallest unit in the written language (Downing, 1973). Blissymbols were originally conceived of as an international

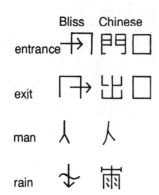

	Bliss	Chinese
entrance		
exit		
man		
rain		

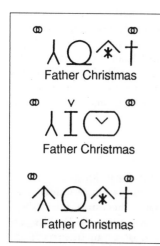

Father Christmas

Father Christmas

Father Christmas

written language, with Chinese as a model. The aim was to promote peace by enabling statesmen from different countries to communicate more easily with one another (Bliss, 1965). The system was never put to such use. It was first used in Toronto as a system of writing for physically disabled children who were unable to speak, and who also had difficulty in learning to read and write (McNaughton and Kates, 1974).

The Bliss system consists of 100 basic signs that can be combined to form words for which there are no basic signs. A number of these sign combinations are conventional – i.e. the Bliss Institute in Toronto and the International Bliss Committee have adopted a fixed English gloss, or 'translation'– but this must be adjusted to fit the national language. A specific sign or a given combination will be used slightly differently in the different countries, in the same way as a word in the spoken language when translated is not exactly the same in another language. Where a conventional combination has not been decided upon, there may be several ways of saying the same word, as can be seen in the example with FATHER CHRISTMAS.

Communication boards with Blissymbols usually consist of both basic signs and the sign combinations that users need frequently. For the majority of words in the spoken languages, however, there are no established conventions, and in many cases users would either not know the accepted form or else not have the necessary basic signs. Thus, it is up to users themselves to find a suitable sign combination to express what they wish to say.

The signs that form a sign combination may be regarded as *semantic elements*. The single signs are combined and understood by analogy. This gives the sign combination meaning. For example, ELEPHANT usually consists of ANIMAL + LONG + NOSE. HOME is HOUSE + FEELINGS. TOILET is CHAIR + WATER. HAPPY is FEELING + UP (Figure 2). In addition to the signs that correspond to whole words, there are also several Blissymbols that constitute grammatical inflections and denote parts of speech, such as PAST, PLURAL, ACTION, OPPOSITE-MEANING, etc. Thus the Bliss system has a fairly complex construction, based on combinations of signs.

The basic signs and sign combinations may also be joined together to form sentences. Bliss (1965) gives information about syntax, but in principle any word order may be used. In most countries the word order resembles the spoken language as closely as possible.

The graphic formation of a number of words can be fairly complex. Additionally, many signs have one or more basic signs in common. For individuals with normal vision and good linguistic and intellectual skills this may not

Figure 2. *Blissymbols.*

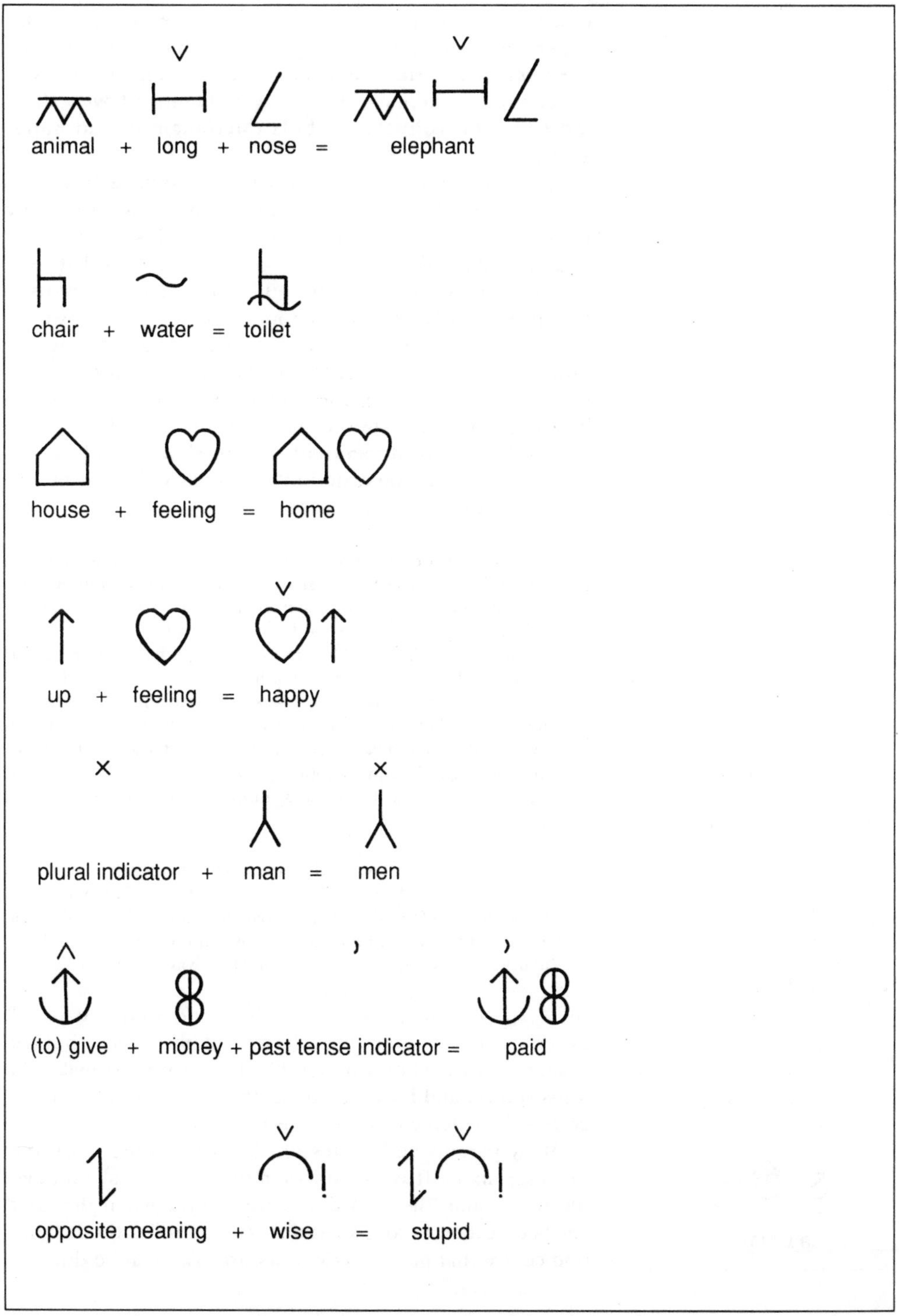

matter, but for severely mentally handicapped individuals this complexity can be a great barrier. With the exception of cases where only the simplest signs have been taught, experiments in teaching Blissymbols to this group have not been very successful. Intellectually competent people with speech impairments and reading difficulties have gained most benefit from Blissymbols (McNaughton and Kates, 1980).

It has sometimes been said that conversational partners who can read do not need to know Blissymbols because the word is always written above the sign. This is true with regard to the basic signs and sign combinations that exist on the communication board. When combinations are used to express words that are not found on the board, however, the listener must know how the system is constructed in order to understand what the user means. The user in turn must understand what the listener is capable of comprehending. Communication can be difficult since the possible combinations are dependent on the signs found on the board. Sentence construction is similarly limited by the availability of signs.

> At a youth seminar a non-reading but intellectually competent 20-year-old boy was given the task of communicating to another person something that did not have anything to do with his immediate situation. This he was to do with the aid of his Bliss board containing 240 signs. He tried to say: 'He who has everything also has his health'. After 20 minutes he had still not made himself understood. The conversation was recorded on videotape and shown the following day to a group of adolescents who themselves used communication aids. It was only after a long period of time and a good many probing questions that the group, which consisted of several Bliss users, understood what the boy had wanted to say.

> An adolescent who used Blissymbols told his teacher at school that MOTHER ALMOST-SAME-AS COCA-COLA. It was only when his mother came to school later that day and explained that she had been angry with him that morning that it was understood that the utterance was intended to mean 'Mum was angry'.

In retrospect it is easy to understand that the youth expressed that 'mother was almost bubbling over', but the example clearly shows how difficult it can be to make the signs suffice, and how creative both the user and the listener must be when conversation is nuanced.

Many parents and professionals have reacted negatively to Blissymbols. It is not uncommon for them to sabotage the use of the Bliss board and use it only when the child has been called in for assessment or control at the habilitation centre that has prescribed its use. This can be due to a

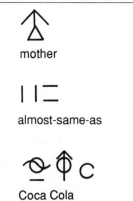

mother

almost-same-as

Coca Cola

lack of introduction to and guidance in the use of the system, and the fact that no explanation has been given as to why Blissymbols have been chosen. For a number of users Blissymbols prove too difficult, and instead of improving communication they lead to frustration both for user and for those close to them. This sometimes happened before other systems had come into use. There are also examples of children being given a Bliss board despite the fact that they could read and write, and would have got greater benefit from a board with letters and words (cf. Conway, 1986; Smith et al., 1989).

PIC

PIC (Pictogram Ideogram Communication) signs originate from Canada (Maharaj, 1980). They have become very popular in the Nordic countries and have, to a great extent, replaced the use of Blissymbols among those with extensive learning difficulties. PIC signs consist of stylised drawings which form white silhouettes on a black background. The gloss is always written in white lettering above the drawing.

PIC signs do not yield the same problems one finds with Blissymbols. Both parents and professionals feel they are easier to understand, and have taken to them quickly. PIC signs are, however, less versatile, and in some respects more limited than Blissymbols. There are only 563 Norwegian PIC signs (1989), and combining them to form new words or sentences is not always easy. When the user needs more opportunities than those given by PIC signs, the signs may be supplemented with signs from other systems which have a more general use.

The use of PIC signs has been of great benefit to many people but their popularity may also have led to overuse,

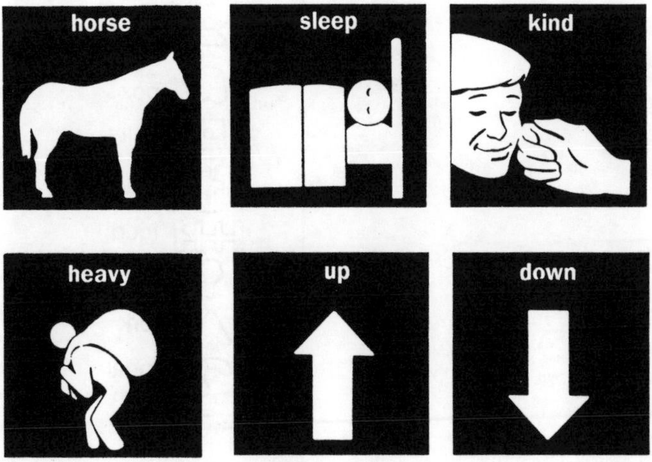

Figure 3. *PIC.*

and they may sometimes have been recommended for people who could have used Blissymbols or normal writing.

Premack's word bricks

Premack's word bricks form a system that has been used fairly extensively in the United Kingdom and the United States for teaching both mentally handicapped and autistic individuals. The word bricks were originally devised in order to investigate whether apes could learn a language that was not based on speech. It was therefore important for Premack (1971) that the word bricks did not resemble those objects they were supposed to represent. This was because he wished to show that apes could learn non-iconic signs. Deich and Hodges (1977) made additional word bricks, and a number of these resemble the objects that they are used to represent. The word bricks are made of plastic or wood and differ in form (Figure 4). What sets these signs apart from others is the fact that they can be physically manipulated and moved.

Premack's system was chiefly aimed at teaching single signs, even though they were also strung together to form

Figure 4. *Premack's word bricks.*

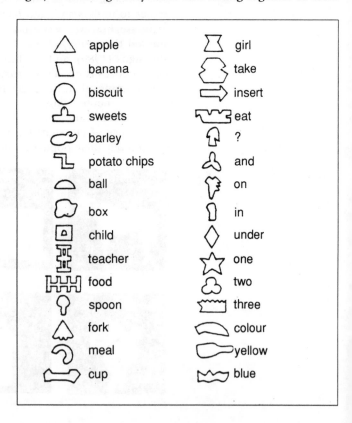

△	apple	⋈	girl
▭	banana	⬚	take
○	biscuit	⇨	insert
⬦	sweets	∿	eat
↻	barley	⋔	?
⌐	potato chips	⋏	and
⌒	ball	⸙	on
▱	box	◊	in
▣	child	◇	under
⬯	teacher	☆	one
⊞	food	♧	two
♀	spoon	∿	three
△	fork	◠	colour
♫	meal	⬭	yellow
⬭	cup	∿	blue

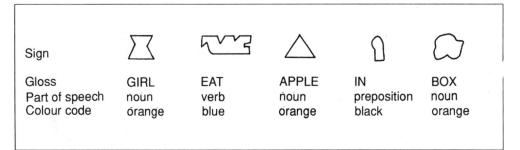

Sign	⏛	ᴎᴍᴤ	△	◊	◯
Gloss	GIRL	EAT	APPLE	IN	BOX
Part of speech	noun	verb	noun	preposition	noun
Colour code	orange	blue	orange	black	orange

Figure 5. *Carrier's sentence building with Premack's word bricks.*

sentences. Carrier developed the use of Premack's word bricks by producing a systematic, pedagogical programme for the teaching of sentence building (Carrier, 1974; Carrier and Peak, 1975). The word bricks were marked with coloured tape to denote the part of speech the word brick belonged to. Articles were marked in red, verbs in blue, nouns in orange, etc. As well as learning how to use single bricks, users would also learn a simplified syntax from the fact that different types of sentences consisted of different colour sequences (Figure 5).

Rebus

As with Blissymbols, the Rebus Reading Series (Woodcock, Clark and Davies, 1969) was devised as a system of logographic writing (Clark, 1984). It was originally made to help people with a lesser degree of mental handicap to learn to read. At a later stage its use was extended to include communication (Jones, 1979). A special version has been made for the UK (van Oosterom and Devereux, 1985; Walker et al., 1985).

The Rebus system is of special interest because to a certain extent it represents a different approach to that of Blissymbols, PIC signs and Premack's word bricks. The system consists of 950 signs, the majority of which are iconic. It is possible to combine these in the usual way: STREET + LIGHT becomes STREETLIGHT (Figure 6). In addition to the usual combinations of words, the pronunciation of the sign's gloss may also be used. For example, LIGHT can mean both 'bright' and 'not heavy'. This is especially useful in English-speaking countries where there are many homonyms.

In teaching Rebus, emphasis is placed on using letters as well as signs. The letters are combined with the pronunciation of the glosses so that the combinations of signs and letters form new words. When a sign is combined with a letter, it is the pronunciation of these two elements together that expresses the new word. The meaning of the sign plays no part. P + LIGHT becomes PLIGHT, S + AT becomes SAT, and H + EAT becomes HEAT (Figure 6).

Figure 6. *Rebus signs.*

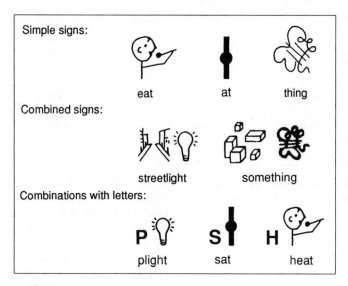

Training in the use of the Rebus system has proved to have a positive effect on the individual's reading skills (Kiernan, Reid and Jones, 1982), and this is related to the practice of using corresponding sounds as well the signs' traditional meanings. At the same time the Rebus system places few demands on reading skills, since it is not necessary to be able to read all the letters in a word. Investigations into the teaching of reading and sound recognition show that initially children are able to say what the first sound or syllable is in a word, without being able to identify the other sounds (Skjelfjord, 1976). Thus, it seems as though the Rebus system is based on a mid-stage in the acquisition of reading skills, and thereby enhances the further development of these skills.

Other sign systems

Lexigrams

Lexigrams do not constitute a complete sign system. They consist of a set of nine elements which may be combined in different forms and assigned glosses (Figures 7 and 8). As there are no fixed or allocated signs, the sign's gloss is assigned on the basis of the needs of each individual. As with Premack's system, the stated aim is that the signs shall not be based on iconicity (Romski, Sevcik and Pate, 1988). Lexigrams have mostly been used in the United States, although their use seems to have been limited to teaching trials.

PCS

Picture Communication System (Johnson, 1981; 1985) consists of approximately 1800 signs. The signs are simple line drawings with the word written above. In some cases, the written word appears without any line drawing (Figure 9). The signs are easy to draw, and PCS can therefore be easily copied by hand. PCS is common in the United States and Spain.

SIGSYM

These signs are based on both iconicity and sign language. The graphic signs that are made from manual signs show characteristics that are typical of the execution of manual signs (Figure 10). Since manual signs differ from country to country and between the various systems, it is essential that the Sigsym signs are designed on the basis of the sign language in use in the particular area. There are, for example, Sigsym signs for British Sign Language (Cregan, 1982) and American Sign Language (Cregan and Lloyd, 1984). Sigsym

Figure 7. *The nine main elements in Lexigrams.*

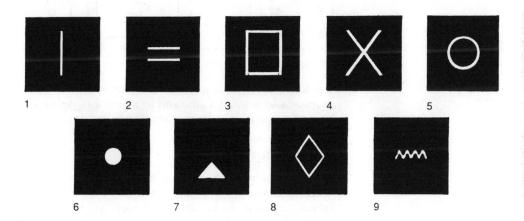

Figure 8. *Examples of Lexigrams.*

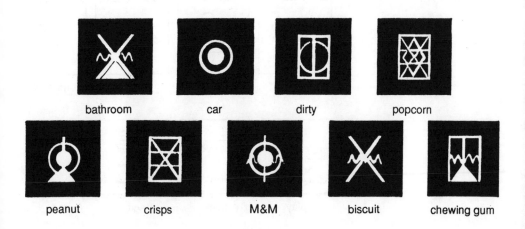

Figure 9. *Picture Communication System.*

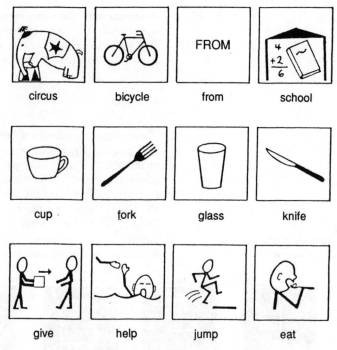

would appear to be of interest for individuals who use both graphic and manual signs, and as a possible written language for people who learn manual signs.

Orthographic script

Many communication aids are based on normal writing. Since spelling out words and sentences letter by letter can take a long time, an aid that uses letters will often contain combinations of letters, words and sentences in addition to single letters. For users who have only a limited vocabulary, the communication aid may consist of single words.

Figure 10. *Sigsym.*

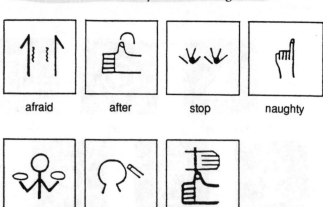

Pictures

Pictures, i.e. drawings and photographs, have commonly been used as a first communication aid. The desire to use something which the individual can recognise and react to is generally the argument used in favour of pictures. However, pictures have both advantages and disadvantages. A *general* interest in pictures may be an argument for using a sign system based on iconicity, providing that the person does not have fixed routines related to the act of 'looking at pictures'. If the individual is interested in *particular* pictures, the use is dependent on what he or she associates with these images. Looking at and reacting to pictures is not a *linguistic use*, and the use of pictures as words may necessitate the individual unlearning his or her original use of such images. Unlearning established reactions to known pictures is the same as removing part of the basis that forms an already existing interaction, and this seems neither necessary nor wise.

Small children show a limited comprehension of pictures (Kose, Beilin and O'Connor, 1983). For example, in early language development the names of learned objects are not transferred to pictures of those same objects (Lucariello, 1987). Picture comprehension is limited among many mentally retarded people too, and photographs may be more difficult to comprehend than line drawings (Dixon, 1981; McNaughton and Light, 1989). If the individual does not understand what the pictures are supposed to represent, then there is little point in using pictures.

Most people are surrounded by pictures, and for those who are to use pictures as 'words', it can be difficult to distinguish between pictures used in the ordinary manner – to look at and remember, to talk about, as decoration and illustrations, etc. – and pictures that form part of the individual's own vocabulary. Using pictures that are distinctive and totally different from others, and defining these as the individual's vocabulary, is therefore helpful. The majority of graphic sign systems are largely based on iconicity, while at the same time they have their own special characteristics that distinguish them from usual pictures (for example, PCS and PIC). It is therefore beneficial to use a graphic sign system instead of pictures.

The use of sign systems may also facilitate naming, which is difficult when a child has to communicate with the aid of pictures. For example, parents and children often sit with picture books and tell each other the names of things they see in them. If the pictures on the communication board are fairly similar to those in the books, there is little purpose in pointing both in the book and at the communication board. This is only a form of matching, and does not

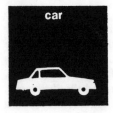

imply a linguistic use. Pointing at the picture on the communication board would be difficult to perceive as naming of the objects and activities in the picture in the book, which is a condition for calling it linguistic use.

In addition, it seems that pictures are not generally regarded as an individual's language. Users experience that they are not taken seriously when they communicate by means of pictures, and that pointing at a picture is not taken as an expression of the fact that they have something to say (Conway, 1986). Parents often act as though the child has merely pointed at an ordinary picture, and may begin to talk about what is in the picture, what is happening in it, etc. (C. Basil, personal communication, 1989).

When making pictures for communication boards, many people use pictures of things the child recognises, and of the child in the situation the picture is used to represent. For example, the parents may take a photograph of their car and try to teach the child to use it as the generic term for 'car'. This may make it difficult for the child to use the picture to talk of cars other than that particular one. The familiarity, which at the outset should be considered an advantage, becomes an obstacle because the picture is treated a proper name – 'Mummy and Daddy's car' – instead of a generic name for a class of objects, 'cars'. Imagine that photographs of a child's mother and father were used as general expressions for 'man' and 'woman', i.e. to speak of all men and women, and the problem becomes even clearer.

Similar problems arise with photographs of the child in the swimming pool, car, gymnasium, etc. The pictures focus attention on the child instead of the situation. Pictures of this type make it difficult to speak of just the swimming pool, or to say that others are in the swimming pool, gymnasium, etc.

Many pictures are also cut out of magazines and placed on the communication board without taking into account how difficult it sometimes is to distinguish between pictures. Some mentally handicapped individuals are either colour blind or unable to utilise colour information (J.F. Fagan, personal communication, 1987). This is one argument in favour of using a sign system in black and white with good contrast, because the likelihood that the user will perceive and comprehend the differences between the signs is greatest in such a system.

Choosing a sign system

In order to find the best form of communication for an individual in need of augmentative communication, it should first be determined whether he or she should begin with an aided or unaided form of communication. A choice must be made between a manual or graphic sign system, or it may be decided to use both systems. Then there is the question of which manual or graphic system to use as a basis.

Comparing different sign systems is not an easy task. Within one country, standardised use may be the most important argument for choosing one system instead of another. It is highly important that as many people as possible use the same system so that it is easier for teachers and other professionals to continue the work with children and adolescents from other schools and institutions. Care should be taken to ensure that the users are able to communicate with one another directly. In Britain this means that it is generally best to stick to British Sign Language and British manual signs, and to the graphic systems that are in general use. Convincing proof of the need for a particular new sign system would be required in order for that sign system to be taken into use. Standardised use also increases the possibilities of gaining broad experience with a system, and thereby revealing its strong and weak points.

Manual or graphic signs

When choosing between manual and graphic signs, the individual's perceptual abilities should be taken into account. Visually impaired individuals can often comprehend the movements of manual signs more easily than they can perceive a drawing. The movements can also be understood kinaesthetically, as in communication among people with a combined visual and hearing impairment where the manual signs of the conversational partner are performed with the user's hands. For some users, technical aids with graphic sign systems and synthetic speech will be helpful. Many mentally disabled people gain little benefit from pictures, but for others graphic signs have a great attention value. Some graphic signs may be physically manipulated (Premack), but little is known of how this may influence learning and use.

The ability to use one's arms and hands is also an important factor in the choice of communication form. One significant difference between manual and graphic signs is the fact that graphic signs are selected while manual signs must be produced. Manual signs therefore appear to place greater demands on memory.

There are a number of circumstances that may be important in the choice between a manual and graphic system, but of which little is known. Assertions about the functional differences between the systems are often based on suppositions.

Few studies have compared aided and unaided communication. The best investigation is that carried out by Hodges and Schwethelm (1984). They compared the learning of manual signs and Premack's word bricks among 52 mentally handicapped children and adolescents (5–17 years) with an average non-verbal IQ score of 13. There were four groups with 13 people in each group. In an initial three-month period, one of the groups was taught to use Premack's word bricks as prescribed by Hodges and Deich (1978). Another group was taught to use the bricks using the method prescribed by Carrier and Peak (1975). The last two groups were not given any training for the first three months. In the next two months, the first two groups, plus one of the others, were taught manual signs (Table 1).

Table 1. *The teaching of Hodges and Schwethelm's groups (1984)*.

Group	First period of training (3 months)	Second period of training (2 months)
1	Training in the use of Premack's word bricks according to the method prescribed by Hodges and Deich (1978)	Training in the use of manual signs
2	Training in the use of Premack's word bricks according to the method prescribed by Carrier and Peak (1975)	Training in the use of manual signs
3	No sign training	Training in the use of manual signs
4	No sign training	No sign training

To begin with, both of the groups that began with the word bricks were trained in matching, and they were taught to use graphic signs only when they had managed the matching tasks. Only seven of the 26 children in these two groups managed the matching tasks and were able to continue with the word bricks. Of the 19 children who were not sufficiently adept at matching, 12 learned from one to 11 manual signs in the second phase. Only one of the children who learned to use word bricks did not learn to use manual signs. Having been taught the use of graphic signs did not appear to have any significance for the use of manual signs. The children in the first two groups learned an average of 4.3 manual signs, while the group that had not been taught during the first three months learned an average of five manual signs.

The experiment reflects not only the difference between manual and graphic signs, but the teaching methods differed as well. Carrier places great emphasis on the matching of colours and numbers as a criterion for learning graphic signs. Hodges and Deich also emphasise skills in matching. The extent to which the matching tasks were accomplished did not, however, prove to be crucial for whether the manual signs were learned or not. It is quite likely that several of the children could have learned to use graphic signs if another, more functional, teaching method had been used. On the other hand, it may be easier to establish a functional teaching situation with manual signs.

Thus, it is difficult to draw reliable conclusions from this experiment. Nonetheless, it does suggest that it is best to begin with manual signs if the individual does not have any special difficulty in using his hands. There are, however, also examples of children who have learned to use aided communication after manual sign teaching had been unsuccessful. One of the children in Hodges and Schwethelm's experiment (1984) learned to use the word bricks but did not learn to use manual signs during the course of the second teaching period. In another experiment (Deich and Hodges, 1977) a 9-year-old boy rapidly learned to use Premack's word bricks, despite the fact that previous manual sign teaching had proved unsuccessful. Later, he also learned to use manual signs. It is conceivable that learning to use word bricks laid the foundations for learning manual signs.

Use of the systems

When factors related to learning do not indicate which sign system is best suited for an individual, other circumstances should be given more emphasis. One of the great advantages of manual signs is that they can be taken everywhere. The individual does not need to carry a board or aid. On the other hand, many graphic signs are easier to understand for people who are unfamiliar with the system. The desire for mobility and a large vocabulary, and the desire to be easily understood by many people, are often contradictory when it comes to choosing augmentative communication. What should be given most priority depends on the individual who will use the system. For a well-functioning adolescent who cannot write, who is in the company of many friends and relations, or who often meets new people, a graphic system may prove to be the most beneficial. For a severely handicapped autistic adolescent who is seldom in contact with people except at home or in a school or institution, manual signs may be the best choice because those with whom he or she is acquainted can be expected to learn the signs, and because the individual will not have to remember to carry a communication board around at all times.

It is not always necessary to choose *between* graphic and manual signs. In some cases graphic signs can supplement the use of manual signs.

> A 13-year-old boy with a moderate intellectual disability learned to use a small communication aid that enabled him to write messages on paper (Memowriter). This he used when he met people who did not know manual signs. He also learned to ask people first in writing whether they knew manual signs. If the answer was positive, he began to use manual signs, which were quicker to use. If the answer was negative, he continued to write. He had approximately the same size vocabulary in manual signs as he did in writing, a little over 300 words (Reichle and Ward, 1985).

> An 8-year-old girl with a minor mental handicap had a good understanding of language but she had great problems expressing herself using speech. She learned to use both manual signs and a communication board with graphic signs. The girl preferred the manual signs but used the board in situations where the manual signs did not suffice (Culp, 1989).

Manual signs

With regard to the sign languages that have been used in the teaching of deaf children, there is no evidence to suggest that one sign language is easier or more difficult to learn than another. All the sign languages have some signs that are easy to perform and others that are more difficult. Those sign systems that follow speech contain the inflections of the spoken language and, if these are included, the signs may become rather complex. Natural sign languages have inflections too. The sign system's degree of difficulty is less dependent on the sign system used than it is on the extent to which inflections are used. In the early stages of teaching the use of inflections is unnecessary.

For individuals with dyspraxia (difficulty in performing intentional actions) or other forms of motor disability, it is advantageous if the signs are simple to perform. In the vast majority of experiments with manual signs, sign systems that were originally designed for deaf children have been used. When necessary, the signs have been simplified so that people with motor disorders would find them easier to perform. This has worked well.

Graphic sign systems

Language comprehension is an important consideration when choosing a graphic sign system. Blissymbols, for example, place greater demands on language comprehen-

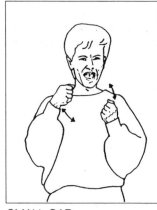

SMALL CAR

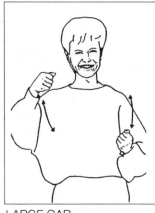

LARGE CAR

sion than PIC signs. These sign systems are also aimed at different groups, i.e. they are intended for people with varying degrees of language comprehension.

There is currently considerable discussion about the characteristics of graphic sign systems, and how easy they are to learn (Clark, 1984; Fuller and Lloyd, 1987). Experiments have predominantly shown that for people without communication disorders Rebus signs are easier to learn than Blissymbols, which in turn are easier to learn than Premack's word bricks (Clark, 1981). Drawings are easier to learn than Blissymbols (Hurlbut, Iwata and Green, 1982). Blissymbols, Premack's word bricks, Rebus signs and Lexigrams are easier to learn than normal writing (Clark, 1981; Romski et al., 1985), but only if the individual is unable to spell. By using normal writing, the individual who is able to spell has access to an unlimited number of words without needing to remember every single one.

It thus appears that there is a certain hierarchy in terms of how difficult the various sign systems are to learn. However, it is not certain that the relative ease of learning is the same for those who use the systems. There are, for example, no comparisons of the use of PIC signs and Premack's word bricks in the teaching of mentally handicapped people. Many of the systems are very similar, and those who claim that one system is better than another often base this on supposition, or make the claim because they have participated in the creation of that particular system. For example, it is conceivable that it is better to use a white silhouette on a black background, as is the case with PIC signs, than it is to use normal line drawings, such as those found in PCS. However, this remains to be demonstrated.

Nor is it the case that the vocabularies of the sign systems are tailor-made for each user. They represent limitations with regard to the signs that can be learned. Even though a good deal of work has gone into choosing the signs that make up an individual system, the vocabulary should nonetheless be regarded as a suggestion. The user's requirements should determine which signs should appear on the communication board, and if a word that is required does not exist, a new sign should be made. In order to emphasise the signs' linguistic function, it may nonetheless be helpful if the home-made signs resemble the sign system the individual uses. There is, for example, no PIC sign for 'finished'. FINISHED has often proved to be a useful manual sign, and one may therefore make a graphic sign consisting of a white silhouette on a black background for people who otherwise use PIC signs. Since lexigrams are also white on black, one of these could possibly be used. With regard to names of people, places, etc., it is often

finished

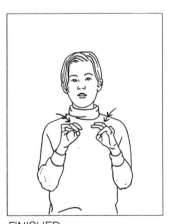

FINISHED

practical to use photographs.

There is no reason to be afraid of mixing different graphic sign systems. There is nothing magical about them that requires one to stick to one system only. PIC signs will, for example, gradually become too limited for many users, and Blissymbols may be placed among the PIC signs as a link in the developmental chain. Blissymbols generally have a wider use than PIC signs, and therefore make a more useful instrument for the user. At the same time, Blissymbols place greater demands on, and build on, the communicative skills which the user has acquired through the use of PIC signs.

Chapter 3
Communication aids

The term *communication aid* is commonly used to denote aids that help users express themselves. Hearing aids are regarded as an aid to the senses, while glasses are not considered an aid in the same way. Neither of these resources is considered to be a communication aid, though, despite the fact that both undoubtedly contribute to improving communication between individuals.

Communication aids have been in use for a long time, and range from 'manual' boards and aids employing simple technology, with, for example, lights and pointers that move, to aids based on advanced computer technology utilising monitors and artificial speech (see Fishman, 1987; Vanderheiden and Lloyd, 1986). Communication aids, and the way they are used, have received increased attention since communication aids employing computer-based technology have come into use.

The ease of access to communication aids is usually most important for people with physical disabilities, but many speech-impaired individuals who are not physically disabled may also benefit from their use. Communication aids should be transportable so that they are accessible in a variety of situations. Technical aids in particular have, until recently been fairly heavy or bulky and therefore difficult to carry around. Some have also required an external power supply. Physically disabled people who are relatively immobile have found it easier to use such aids than other, more mobile, individuals. Users of electric wheelchairs have been able to plug the aids into the wheelchair battery. Relatively heavy, battery-driven communication aids may be easy to transport with the help of a wheelchair, but are little help to users if they have to be carried. Individuals who do not need wheelchairs will therefore tend to use more traditional pointing boards or books with graphic signs or pictures.

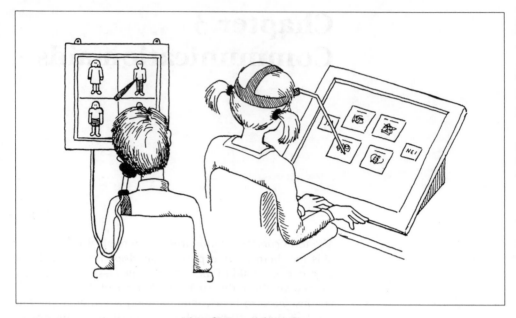

Figure 11. *Examples of traditional aids.*

Traditional aids

Traditional aids are generally boards or trays with letters, words, graphic signs or pictures (Figure 11). In some cases the board may contain only numbers or another form of *code* that refers to a list of words (glossary). A number code, or its equivalent, gives users the means of expressing a greater number of words, signs or sentences than they would otherwise be able to reach.

The aids are controlled with the help of *direct selection* and *automatic* or *directed scanning*.

Direct selection means that the user points directly at what he or she wants to say. The pointing may be done with a finger, a foot, a pointing-stick attached to the head, a beam of light, the eyes, etc.

Automatic scanning implies that a light, a pointer, or something similar moves. The user activates some form of switch when the light or pointer is in the desired position.

Directed scanning is usually performed when the user activates two or more switches. One or more switches are used to move a beam of light, pointer, etc., around the board and another switch is used to make the selection.

Directed and automatic scanning can be either simple or combined.

Simple scanning describes the process whereby all the signs on the board are scanned in rotation (Figure 12).

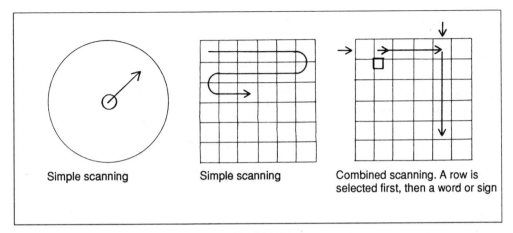

Simple scanning   Simple scanning   Combined scanning. A row is
                                               selected first, then a word or sign

Figure 12. *Simple and combined scanning.*

Combined scanning implies that each dimension is scanned separately. This may, for example, mean that the individual selects a row first, and then selects the sign in the row he or she wants to look at. There are, however, several ways of organising the scanning (Figure 12).

When the user has a large vocabulary, simple scanning can be very time-consuming. Combined scanning is quicker and more effective. With small children and mentally retarded individuals, it is natural to begin with simple scanning and progress to combined scanning when the simple scanning has been mastered.

There are also dependent and independent forms of scanning.

Independent scanning means that the user directs or stops the scanning pointer, for example a light without help from anyone else.

Dependent scanning means that another person (the helper) points systematically at the board and the user indicates when the helper is pointing at the desired row, letter, word or sign by uttering a sound, blinking, etc.

Direct selection requires that the individual has relatively good motor coordination and reach. Directed scanning demands that the user is able to carry out repeated movements, while automatic scanning requires that the user can coordinate his or her own movements with the movements of a light, pointer, etc. An individual is more sensitive than a technical aid. Dependent scanning can therefore be a good way of starting a more varied form of communication with children who are dependent on scanning, but who are at present incapable of mastering an independent scanning technique. In situations where it is impossible to find a movement that the individual can utilise, dependent scan-

> GOOD PEOPLE ARE
> ALWAYS HAPPY
> *KARINA*

> JESPER THE COWARD
> SHUTS HIS BODY AND
> SOUL CAN'T OPEN THEM
> NOT EVEN WITH
> WITH HELP AND ONE
> DAY I WILL CHOOSE MY
> OWN LIFE
> *JESPER*

> I SLEEP ON THE SOFA ALL
> DAY WITH BEANS IN MY
> BELLY
> *KARL*

> NOW YOU HAVE YOUR
> DOUBTS
> *KARSTEN*

> I DON'T WANT TO BE
> STERILISED BECAUSE
> THAT MEANS AN
> OPERATION. I'VE USED
> THE PILL BEFORE SO I'D
> LIKE TO USE IT AGAIN
> *MAJA*

> OUR FRIENDSHIP IS
> GOOD
> KARIN IS ALSO MY
> FRIEND
> *LEO*

> LOVE BETWEEN FRIENDS
> IS DIFFERENT
> I CAN'T EXPLAIN IT
> LOVE BETWEEN ADULTS
> IS GREATER THAN
> INFATUATION
> *PERNILLE*

ning is also useful. A change in facial expression or posture may well be enough if the helper knows the user well. The general objective, though, should always be that the scanning gradually becomes independent.

In Denmark a dependent form of direct selection has caused a great deal of debate. A group of severely disabled youths at a home for mentally disabled people proved able to use letter boards when they were given help with the pointing. They were unable to speak or use sign language, nor were they able to point at the letters on the board on their own. When helped, they were not only able to give voice to their needs, but also to advanced thoughts and feelings toward other residents, their family and staff (Bo-enheden M-huset, 1986). There are, however, many people who do not believe that the residents themselves have done the writing. They claim that the helpers have done it and feel that this point of view is strengthened by the fact that not everyone is able to help the users to write. The controversy continues, but it is in any case possible to imagine that the residents in 'House M' are so dyspractic, i.e. have such extensive motor disorders, that they require a great deal of sensitive help in order to be able to point at what they want. They become dependent on people who can give them such sensitive help and are unable to use technical aids that are less sensitive.

Traditional communication aids, i.e. manual and 'low-tech' aids, are used a lot and fulfil important functions for many users. However, they do have a number of weaknesses. Using a letter board is time-consuming if the listener does not guess the words and sentences correctly before the user has finished spelling. It may take several minutes for the user to point at the letters that make up a single word or wait for an automatic scanning device to move to the desired sign or letter. When the user produces long utterances, it is easy for the communication to break down because the listener has difficulty in retaining the words spoken earlier while simultaneously registering the letters in the next word. It may also be difficult to concentrate on what the user is doing. In ordinary conversation the listener may divert his or her gaze without this causing problems in following what has been said. In a conversation with someone who uses traditional aids, a little inattentiveness can lead to bad guesswork and frustration, and the user's utterance may be either not understood or misunderstood.

New-generation aids

New-generation aids are often based on computer technology. For a while it was common to use special programs on a personal computer which could also be used for educational purposes, work, play and entertainment. Unfortunately, it is impossible to use programs specially designed for one type of machine on another system: for example, Apple, BBC and IBM computers all use different operating systems. In time, more suitable programs will probably become available for IBM-compatible or Macintosh machines, but, as of 1990, it is still BBC and Apple computers that have the best selection of software for small children and individuals with relatively severe mental disabilities.

Ordinary computers are, however, used less and less as an aid to replace the function of speech (Beukelman, 1986). Instead, dedicated communication aids based on computer technology have been produced. These can be transported with relative ease, at least by wheelchair users, and are specifically designed for the tasks they are required to perform.

Ordinary personal computers are designed to be used in many ways, and the fact that they are so widespread is a significant factor in the development of computerised communication functions. This applies especially to their use in nursery schools, schools, at work, or at home for writing essays, letters, orders, tax returns, poetry, etc. Many individuals who use graphic signs have never written a letter by themselves, and a computer with graphic signs can provide them with a whole new realm of opportunities. This applies not only to intellectually competent individuals. Mentally handicapped individuals with some writing skills (ordinary writing or graphic signs) can enjoy sending letters with birthday greetings, messages, etc.

> Ken is a 12-year-old boy with cerebral palsy and a moderate degree of mental handicap. He is unable to speak, but has a good understanding of language. He uses a few manual signs and a communication board with 25 Rebus signs. He cannot write. When he was given the opportunity to use a computer with a concept keyboard, it took no time at all before he began writing letters, especially to his girlfriend (Figure 13).

In order for a user of graphic signs to operate a personal computer, there must be a computer program available for the sign system being used. There are relatively few computer programs available that use sign systems, although programs that employ the most commonly used sign systems, Blissymbols and PIC signs, are available for most types of computer system (e.g. Apple, BBC, Commodore Amiga, IBM). However, not all these programs are user-friendly. In particular, individuals with autism or mental disabilities, including those with a good command of the sign system in question, may have difficulty in using them.

In addition to their use as communication aids, computers can be programmed to function as environmental

Figure 13. *A letter written by a*
mentally handicapped boy
(Osguthorpe and Chang, 1987).

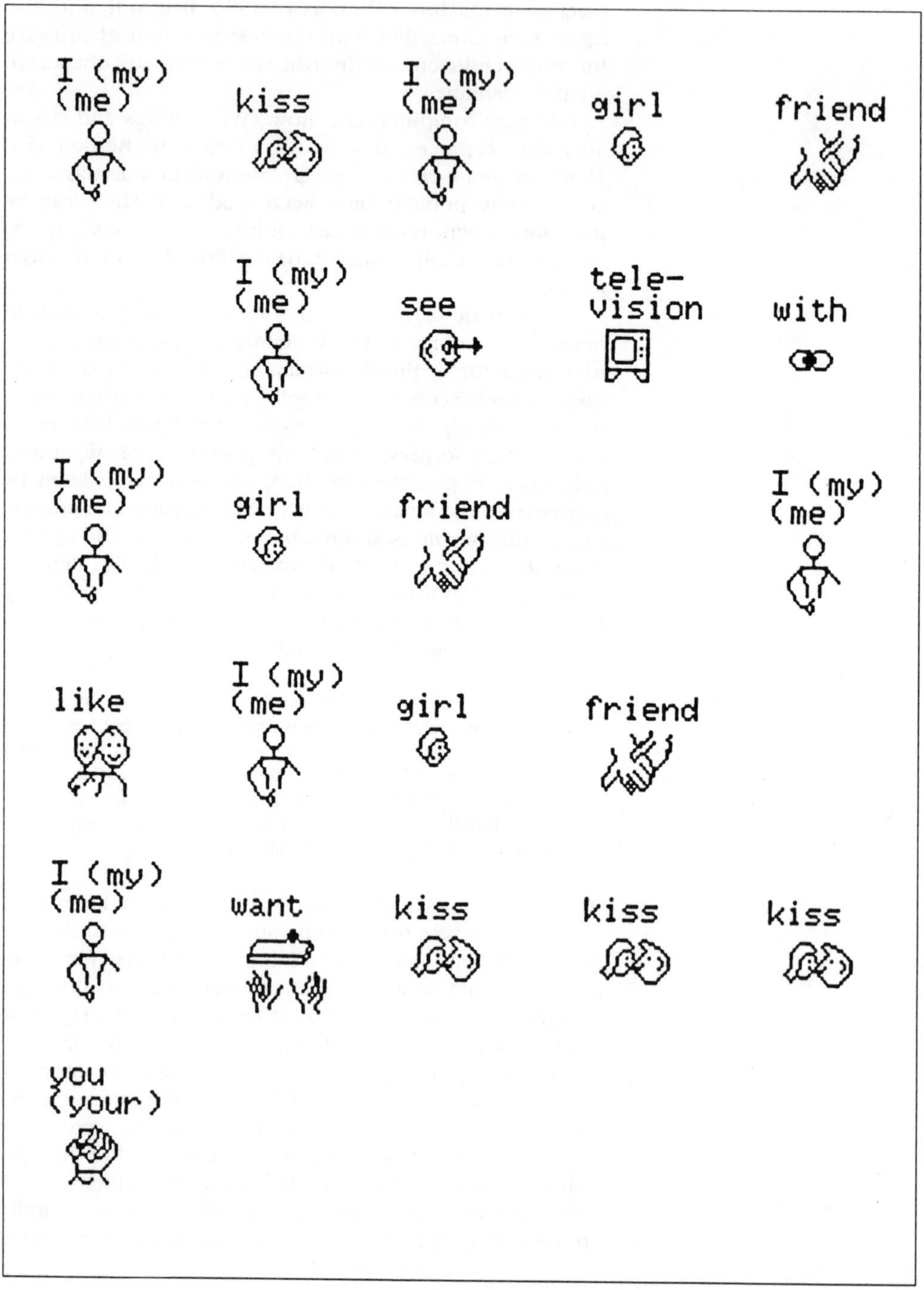

controls, i.e. they may be used to open doors, turn the radio, television, and lights on and off, turn pages in a book, etc. Computers can also be used for other educational purposes, and for playing games. Games that can be controlled with the aid of switches can have a special significance for children with severe motor disorders. *Aided play* provides opportunities for independent activity, and gives disabled children and their caregivers a common interest and something to talk about. In addition, the games can help train skills that may be used later in communicative situations. For example, the BBC program 'Where is Blob' is a variation on the game of hide-and-seek, where the child can make a partially hidden animal appear by activating a switch. Once this has been learned, the child can select an animal by pressing the switch when a star shines above the animal that he or she wishes to appear (Figure 14). It is easy to see how this game – and the scanning skills – can encourage functional language acquisition.

Synthetic speech is common in many computer games, especially American ones. These games can be good fun, and this is a good reason for playing them. But if the aim is to improve the communication skills of a disabled child, then one should be aware that a game that utilises synthetic speech will not in itself improve the child's ability to communicate. True enough, the games do 'speak', but they are

Figure 14. *Blob is as switch-controlled program for BBC computers. A star moves over three animals that are partially hidden behind a wall. When the child presses a switch, the animal below the star appears.*

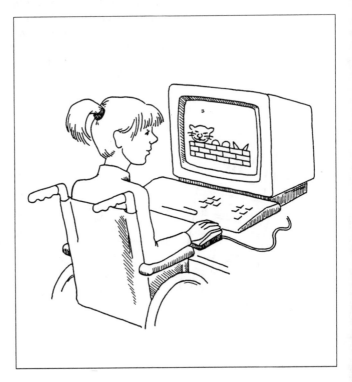

not engaged in a dialogue with the child. What is being said has no functional significance, and instead of fostering communicative skills, the stereotyped computer utterances encourage the passive communicative style one encounters among many individuals with motor disorders.

Although ordinary computers have the advantage that they can be used for a variety of activities, one definite disadvantage of using them as communication aids is that the individual is unable to communicate while using the computer to do other things. Many such activities require a good deal of communication, so it is important that the individual has a means of communicating while doing them. This emphasises the limitations of aids that have too many functions, and shows how essential it is to have a specialised communication aid, even though this may well be more limited in function or vocabulary than an ordinary personal computer.

As with the traditional aids, new-generation communication aids are based on direct selection and scanning. However, they are more flexible. For example, using a computer makes it easy to scroll through pages and gain access to a large vocabulary. If the presentation is visual, then what is being said will remain on screen until it is erased. New-generation aids therefore place fewer demands on the listener's attention (Figure 15). This may make the user and the listener less tense and improve the communicative situation. It will also be easier for the conversational partner to observe non-verbal behaviour, such as facial expressions and posture, without losing the gist of the conversation.

Figure 15. *Examples of newer aids.*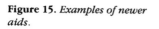

A number of aids that are based on orthographic writing make use of abbreviations or prediction.

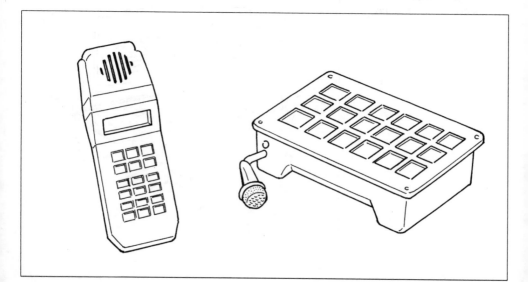

Abbreviations mean that the user only needs to write a couple of letters and then press the space bar or another key in order to spell out the whole word or expression. For example, the user writes *pls*, and *please* will appear on the screen. Abbreviations fill the same function as the combination of letters, words and sentences on manual letter boards. The user may also be able to select a 'word list' after writing one or more letters. Commonly used words that begin with the letters the user has written will then appear on screen, and the user will be able to select the desired word (Figure 16).

Prediction means that the machine makes suggestions as to what the next word or the rest of the word the user is writing will be. If the suggestion is wrong, the user merely continues writing. If the suggestion is correct, he or she can carry on to the next word by typing a full stop, or pressing the space bar, etc. The suggestions are based on the words the user has previously utilised. The machine remembers which words are used, and suggests the word that is most commonly used and that begins with the letter the user has selected. For example, after *f* the machine might suggest *family*, after *fr from* and after *fri Friday*. If *Friday* is the word the user was thinking of, the effort of typing or selecting the letters will have been halved. In some programs several alternatives will appear, and the user may either choose one of these or continue typing.

Abbreviations and prediction can be useful, but both systems are dependent on the words being fairly long and being used often enough for the system to save time. Time is saved on the number of keys pressed, and it has been shown that some of the prediction systems save between 40 and 60 per cent on the number of keystrokes (Balkom, Blom and Soede, 1987; Beukelman, Yorkston and Dowden, 1985). Individuals who type quickly will be interrupted in

Figure 16. *MAC-Apple is a switch-controlled program for Apple II. It can also be used to communicate over the telephone network with the aid of a modem.*

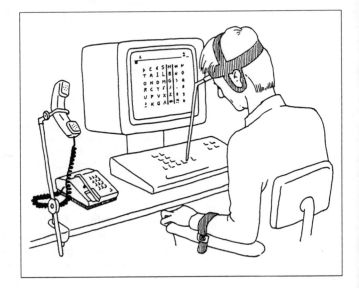

their writing if they have to follow closely what is happening on the screen. For those who type slowly but are quick to follow what is happening on the screen, however, a considerable amount of time can be saved.

Artificial speech

The most important technological developments in new-generation communication aids lie in the use of artificial speech. There are two forms of artificial speech: synthetic and digitised.

> *Synthetic speech* comprises a set of rules for the transferral of combinations of letters to speech (text-to-speech). These rules differ depending on the language spoken, and every country must therefore have its own system. There are several different English systems in use.

An aid that utilises synthetic speech is able to say everything the user writes, but the user must be able to spell and write reasonably quickly in order for the communication to work. Synthetic speech may, however, function well in combination with abbreviations, word lists and predictive systems. Synthetic speech is therefore especially useful for people with good linguistic skills, as it opens up the use of a flexible language and an unlimited vocabulary.

At the present time synthetic speech gives the user few opportunities to vary it and create a distinctive voice. Some systems have a male and a female voice, as well as a child's voice but, for technical reasons, the male voice is more distinct and easier to understand than the others. The child's voice is particularly bad, often sounding like Donald Duck. In general, synthetic speech is more difficult to understand than natural speech but, with regular use, one becomes accustomed to it, just as one might to another regional accent.

> *Digitised speech* is speech that is recorded by people with the aid of a sound sampler and stored in the memory of a computer or other computerised device – for example, a talking aid. A sound sampler is a device that converts sound waves (an analogue signal) to numbers (a digital signal). The speech is stored in this digitised form. Digitised speech is similar to a recording made by a tape recorder, but there is no need to spool backwards or forwards in order to find the word one wishes to say. Digitised speech is therefore better suited than tape recordings for use in talking aids. Digitised speech is not language dependent.

Quite a number of aids based on digitised speech have appeared, but they are still relatively expensive. The advantages of digitised speech are good quality and the possibility of recording a voice that suits the user in terms of dialect, age, sex, etc. The disadvantage of digitised speech is limited vocabulary; each word must be pre-recorded. A sentence may be strung together by selecting several single words, but if it is to have any kind of intonation, the whole sentence must be recorded as one entity.

The use of artificial speech has positive social consequences because conversation becomes more normal. The user does not have to wait to attain eye contact with the listener, or ring a bell, etc. He or she can interrupt and begin speaking in the same way as the other participants in the conversation, hears immediately hear what he or she has said, can verify that the word selected was the right one, and correct any mistakes. Another important advantage is that artificial speech makes it easier for users of communication aids to communicate with one another.

Telecommunication aids - *talking on the telephone*

Practically all language teaching has been directed at face-to-face communication. In society in general, telecommunications play an increasingly important role, and new services are being established. The telephone plays an important role in the maintenance of social networks and the coordination of activities. This is especially true in the activities of young people.

New technology has led to new advanced telephone services and, in addition, the transferral of data has made telecommunication possible for a number of people who previously had no access to it. A speech-impaired individual is able to speak on the telephone using synthetic speech, or transfer text and graphic signs with the aid of a personal computer or text-telephone (Figure 16). There are also aids that make it easier, or even unnecessary, to lift the receiver, that dial the number automatically, etc. Videotelephones, which enable the transferral of live images over the telephone network, will soon be widely available. Thus, it will be possible to communicate over great distances using manual signs. For mentally handicapped individuals, it may be crucial for their understanding of telecommunication equipment that they are able see the person with whom they are communicating.

Paradoxically enough, those groups that are not particularly mobile and who have difficulty visiting others will also have the least opportunity to use telecommunication equipment. As access to telecommunications improves, individuals with language and communication disabilities will have more opportunities to take part in a wider social network. This is especially important for mentally handicapped people now that many of the larger institutions are being closed down in favour of smaller communities, which will mean that the former residents of those institutions will live further apart. Little thought has been given to how those social networks that have been built up over the years spent living in one institution are to be maintained, and how new social networks should be created for those residents who arrive in a small community without having first lived in a large institution. Most mentally handicapped individuals have ordinary relations with other people. They have close friends, with whom they may perhaps live, and other friends and acquaintances whom they would like to see now and again.

When organising communication situations, it is also important to take into account the needs individuals have for telecommunications and the opportunities they represent. These can be extremely important, especially for young people who have left home or are away from their family for long periods of time.

Pointing

Direct selection is often based on touching, pressing buttons or keyboards, etc. or some other form of pointing. Pointing does not necessarily imply the use of an outstretched forefinger. Many individuals with motor disabilities are unable to extend their forefinger, or to use it to point at all. It is important not to be formalistic, but instead to accept the form of pointing the user can manage.

Figure 17. *Different forms of pointing.*

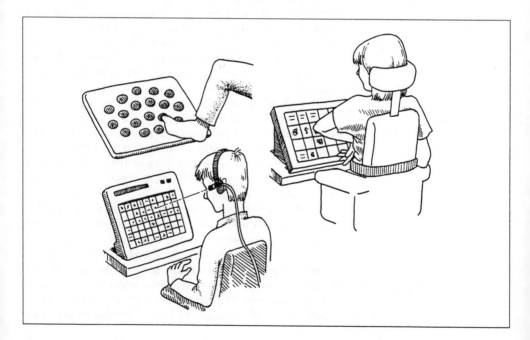

Peter is a 30-year-old severely disabled man. He often experienced problems making himself understood because the staff at his school insisted that he use his forefinger to point at the communication board. It was far easier for him to use the lower joint of his thumb, something that was also accepted at home. By their inflexibility, the school hindered Peter's language acquisition and caused him unnecessary frustration.

For people who are unable to use their hands to point, there are a number of other possibilities. The feet can be a good alternative, or a head stick or a lamp that sends out a beam of light (Figure 17).

A large number of different forms of *eye-pointing* exist for those who have insufficient control over their body or head. There are special coding systems based on eye-pointing (ETRAN), but eye-pointing may also be used in the same way as other forms of pointing (Figure 18). In addition, there are aids that register the direction in which the eye is looking, and that write or say which object a user looks at for longer than, say, three seconds. These forms of eye-pointing are, however, very tiring to use.

Eye-pointing is often considered as a last resort, despite the fact that this form of pointing is a natural part of the communication repertoire of many disabled children. However, there is a difference between an individual who has this as the sole form of expression, and one who simply uses it to point at objects in the environment. Moreover, it is easier to follow eye movement over longer rather than shorter distances.

Figure 18. *Eye-pointing.*

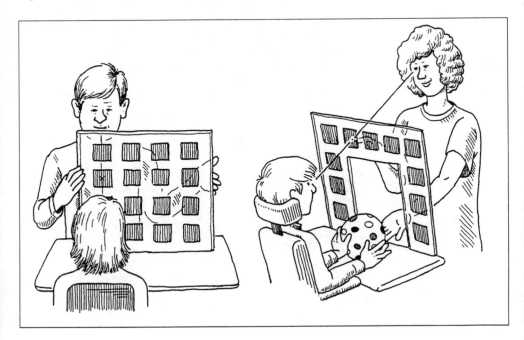

When an individual uses the eyes to point at some kind of board, the conversational partner must be located so that he or she is able to follow the user's gaze, thus dictating how successful the communicative situation will be. Furthermore, the eyes have so many other functions that it is an advantage if another form of pointing can be used. If the user is able to use a hand or foot, it may be easier for the conversational partner to see the pointing. For people who are unable to use their hands or point in other ways, as is often the case with girls with Rett's syndrome, eye-pointing can nonetheless be an effective way for them to state their wishes.

Keyboards

The most common way of utilising a computer is by means of a keyboard. Many communication aids also use ordinary keyboards with letter keys, and in some circumstances extra keys for special functions as well. For people who are unable to reach very far, there are miniaturised keyboards, and for individuals whose aim is fairly inaccurate, there are keyboards with larger keys and more space between each key (Figure 19).

From the time computers began to be used as communication aids, special forms of keyboards called *concept keyboards* have been utilised. A concept keyboard is made up of areas that may be pressed. There are also concept keyboards where the different areas are scanned and one or more of the areas is lit up. The number of areas that can be pressed may vary, but 128 is the usual number. However, several areas may be combined to produce a larger area where all the keys within that one area share the same function. The size of the *functional* fields is therefore not fixed, but depends instead on the program that is in use. If all the keys have the same function, then there will only be one

Figure 19. *Examples of keyboards with different designs.*

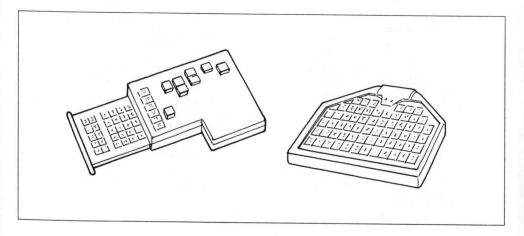

functional field. A concept keyboard with 128 keys may thus have between 1 and 128 functional fields. By giving several keys the same function, it is easy to adjust the concept keyboard to a individual's motor and linguistic ability. The keys are covered with a sheet of paper on which the functional fields are marked off. These may consist of letters, words, signs, pictures, etc. (Figure 20). On both ordinary computer keyboards and concept keyboards it is possible to regulate the sensitivity of the keys. Normally a letter or sign will be repeated if the key is held down, but this function can be turned off so that the pressure on the key must be released before that key is activated again. It is also possible to extend the time the key may be held down before it is reactivated, so that the letter or sign is only repeated after the key has been pressed for, say, two seconds.

The normal operation of a computer often requires that the operator is able to press two keys at the same time. This is difficult or impossible for individuals who have poor coordination skills, are only able to use one hand, or use a head stick. However, there are therefore special programs that enable the user to press keys in sequence to perform a function that normally requires two or more keys to be depressed simultaneously.

Switches

With the use of scanning devices, switches are often activated in order to control the aid. Usually there are one or two switches, but there are also systems that use as many as eight. However, the functional difference between five or eight switches is minimal. When many switches are employed, the difference between keyboards and concept keyboards diminishes. A concept keyboard is in principle a collection of switches that are activated when they are

Figure 20. *Concept keyboards.*

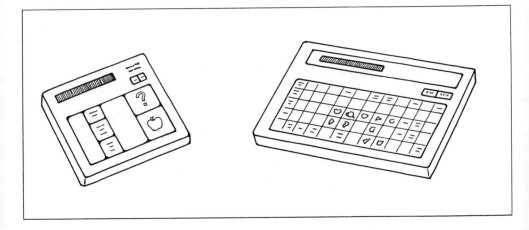

pressed. A switch may be controlled with the hand, arm, foot, head, eyes, etc. There are switches that require little pressure, and switches that can be treated roughly. Switches may be large or small. They can be shaped like a normal light switch, have a 'tongue' through which the hand slips, or consist of a frame that the hand is pushed into. Switches may be activated by sucking and blowing, or by small contractions of the muscles. Some switches consist of a tube containing a drop of mercury that reacts to small positional changes. If the user has better limb control, a joystick or something similar can also be used as a switch. (For an overview of switches and instructions on how to make your own, see Fishman, 1987; Johannessen and Preus, 1989a, 1989b; York, Nietupski and Hamre-Nietupski, 1985).

Using the eyes to activate switches places greater demands on the user than normal eye-pointing. When the eyes are used to activate switches, it is often because it not possible for the user to achieve control of the switches in any other way.

There are two main types of eye switches. The first type consists of a pair of glasses that transmit weak infrared rays to the eye. The rays react to colour changes between the white of the eye and the coloured area (iris). Moving the eye therefore has the effect of turning a switch on or off. The second type of eye switch consists of electrical sensors that are attached behind the eyes. These detect electrical activity in the nerve when impulses from the brain make the eyes move. When the brain sends a message to the eyes telling them to move left and right, the effect is the same as though a switch or two had been flicked.

Figure 21. *Examples of switches and joysticks.*

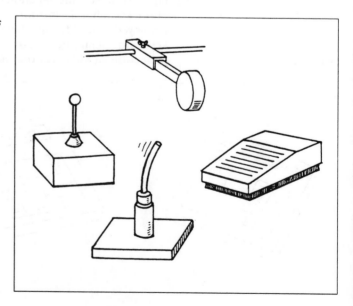

The choice of switches can determine how well an aid will be mastered. There are many different types of switches, but adjusting them is often still the most difficult and time-consuming part of the work of adapting a communication aid for use by individuals with extensive motor disorders. It is very common to begin with the hand, since this seems most 'natural', and go on to try other parts of the body after a long period of training without results. Experience shows that 80 per cent of users have best control of their heads and will most effectively learn to use a head switch first. The hand or foot will often be the first choice for a second switch. Although it is desirable that the individual is able to use a hand, it is more important to make a start by using the aid and avoiding frustration. In cases where hand functions are doubtful, the best strategy is to begin by using the head to activate the switch. If the individual later proves to have good hand control, then it is possible to change to a hand-controlled switch.

A switch that the individual has great difficulty in mastering should not be used. The user may tire quickly, and concentrate more on activating the switch than on the process of communication. It may be advantageous to master several types of switches. The user's general condition will vary from day to day, and it is therefore important to offer the chance of changing to a different type of switch to a user who is tired of using the regular switch.

Choosing a communication aid

Whether the communication aid is to be used on its own or in combination with manual signs, the aim is to find one or several aids that best fill the communication needs the individual has at the moment and in the not too distant future. The communication aids should give the individual the chance to develop. This means that one aid may not always be sufficient. It is also important that the individual feels comfortable using them.

It is usual to begin by assessing the individual's communication needs, list the aids that are suitable, and, by a process of elimination, find the most suitable aid. However, the communication needs will only partially determine the type of communication aid. Most individuals would like to be able to communicate with people who can and cannot read (adults and children) in different situations and in different places. The general objective when educating individuals with communication disorders is to develop these kinds of communication skills. The need to be able to write letters, essays, reports, etc., will vary, but the need for a personal computer for written work should to a certain extent be considered independently of the needs for face-to-face communication. However, the individual's ability to use normal writing will be important for the choice of aid because spelling skills give access to synthetic speech and an unlimited vocabulary.

It is essential to distinguish between the selection of sign system and the selection of an aid. The communication needs, as they appear through an assessment of the individual and the environment in which he or she lives (see the chapter on assessment), will often have more significance for the choice of sign system than the choice of aid. The choice of aid will depend on the individual's physical, linguistic and intellectual abilities, the physical design of the aid, how it is to be transported and used, and how easy it is to learn to use. In cold climates, for example, equipment must function under extremes of temperature and in rain and snow. For a user on holiday in the Mediterranean, a communication aid has to be able to withstand direct sunlight and extremely high temperatures. The priorities one often has to make when choosing an aid reflect the fact that aid development is still in its infancy. These priorities will limit communication, both for intellectually competent people and for mentally handicapped individuals.

One main problem with communication aids is that they are generally designed for use by older children and adults. No communication aids are especially designed for use by children at an age when children generally learn to speak. This means that it is difficult to make provisions for the early development of language skills among children who grow up with aided communication.

Mobility

Mobility is an important factor for everyone who uses communication aids. The aim should be for an individual to have access to as large a vocabulary as possible at any given time. People who use electric wheelchairs can use fairly large and heavy aids. For children and individuals who can walk but are unsteady on their feet, it is essential that the communication aid is not too heavy or bulky. A book containing graphic signs or writing, or a thin board with signs or writing on both sides, may be the best choice for this group, depending on the size of their vocabulary. The problem of transporting aids may make it necessary to have several. A child may have a computer with a large vocabulary, synthetic speech and the possibility of printing at home and in the classroom, and use a pointing board or a small, lightweight aid with digitised or synthetic speech in the school playground and outdoors.

The fact that an aid must be used in many different situations means that the user will not always be seated in a

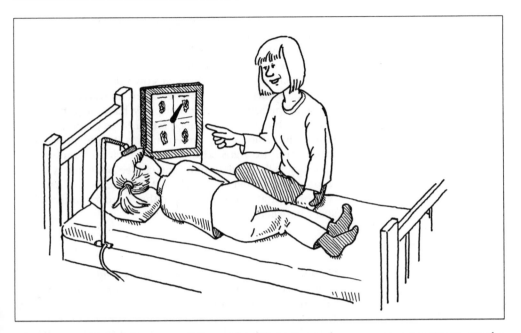

Figure 22. *Communication aids can also be used from a prone position.*

chair or wheelchair. It may be necessary or easier to use the aid when lying down, and it should be possible to alter the aid for such use (Figure 22).

Direct selection and scanning

It is quicker and easier to use direct selection rather than scanning, but the way the individual uses his or her limbs will determine which pointing system should be used. Scanning may be carried out using one or more switch; and the more switches one uses, the less difference there is between direct selection and scanning. The difference between using a joystick and direct selection can in actual fact be fairly small. A joystick has the advantage that it can be adjusted to the individual's motor function by increasing resistance in order to stabilise it so that they amount of force exerted makes no difference. However, a joystick places fairly large demands on motor control and sense of direction.

The choice of direct selection and scanning is determined by the individual's reach, accuracy when pointing, speed, ability to perform several controlled movements successively and activation strength.

Reach and accuracy

Direct selection assumes that the individual is able to reach a sufficient number of signs or letters. For example, people with muscular diseases often have an extremely limited reach. This can be remedied by using such technical aids as a miniaturised keyboard. Scanning with switches or a joy-stick is another way of increasing the individual's functional reach. The beam of light, the pointing stick, etc., functions as an extension of the individual's own direct pointing.

Direct selection also assumes a certain degree of accuracy. Many people with cerebral palsy have no difficulty in reaching things, but they need rather large graphic signs or letters since motor impairment makes it difficult for them to indicate the signs so that they are clearly understood. Accuracy will also determine the choice of switch type and the distance between switches. A low degree of accuracy will necessitate large fields for the switches and a lot of space between them.

Speed

Communicating with aids always takes longer than natural speech, and the aim should always be for the communication to be as quick as possible. Although scanning is a slow method, direct selection is an even slower process for some individuals, and can be more exhausting as well. If it takes a long time from the time a movement is begun until it is completed, scanning may be an alternative because the individual can utilise the time spent scanning to begin his or her own movement. The individual's speed will also determine the scanning rate of the aid, i.e. how quickly the indicator moves from one sign to another.

Repeated movements

Directed scanning can be quicker than automatic scanning provided that the individual is able to carry out several movements in rapid succession. Some people spend a long time preparing themselves, while others are able to carry out several movements in quick succession. Some individuals have problems in stopping after pressing a key the correct number of times. In such cases automatic scanning may be more functional. With technical aids, it is possible to program delays and prevent the user from double-keying by allowing the switch to react only after a certain period of time has passed.

Activation strength

When the signs or text is pointed at, no demands are made on activation strength. If it is necessary to activate switches, press keys or use a concept keyboard in order to display letters or signs on a screen or produce synthetic speech, this requires a certain amount of strength on the part of the user. The various types of keyboards and switches place different demands on activation strength. For a number of aids, the strength required is fairly small, while others require considerably more. For aids that use a keyboard or switches, the individual's activation strength will play an important role in the choice of aid, switch and keyboard.

Manual and technical aids

In discussions of principles for choosing communication aids, a distinction is often made between manual and technical aids. This distinction is not particularly productive, however. It is important to find one or more aids that can enable the individual to communicate. Whether or not a technical aid is used is determined by many different circumstances. A large vocabulary may require an aid based on computer technology. Use of independent scanning will always imply some form of technical device.

It is sometimes claimed that in order to be able to use a technically advanced communication aid, the individual must first have mastered a manual communication aid. There is little basis for this viewpoint. Rather there is reason to believe that the individual who has learned to use a technical aid can also use a manual board with direct selection or dependent scanning if the need should arise, for example, in the case of technical faults or problems with the power supply.

Artificial speech

Artificial speech has chiefly been used in aids for intellectually competent older children, adolescents and adults. Being able to hear the word spoken at the same time as they select a graphic sign or picture may also, however, be of considerable importance for small children and mentally handicapped individuals. The language comprehension the individual has is utilised fully, and understanding of the activity that is taking place may be improved. For an individual with visual impairment, artificial speech may provide crucial cues. The possibility of comparing one's own 'speech' with what others say can facilitate the acquisition of new words. Artificial speech may therefore be more important for individuals in the early stages of language development than for those who have already developed some communication skills.

For individuals with limited language comprehension, it is especially vital that the aid is easy to use; i.e. that there is no need for a long period of training before the aid has a functional use. This is not the same as saying that the aid should be technically simple. An aid utilising artificial speech may be simpler to learn than a manual board because the relationship between the user's actions and the consequences of those actions is made clear.

Price

Many of the newer technical aids are very expensive. This is not an argument against using them, of course, but the usefulness of such aids should be in keeping with their price. Some of them have limited communicative benefit. For a child who communicates quickly and easily with Blissymbols, an aid that employs digitised speech does not necessarily mean an improvement in communication if that aid is difficult to carry around. On the other hand, if the child has not yet learned to read, an aid employing synthetic speech may be of benefit because it provides a chance to use the communicative skills that are being learned. Aids that are difficult to transport are generally rather less expensive than more mobile equipment. These can be used both at home and at school, and the synthetic speech may prove to be essential if the user has difficulty in learning to read.

Some characteristics of communication aids

In order to be a good conversational partner or person in charge of teaching people how to use communication aids, it is vital to know about the special characteristics of aided communication, i.e. how conversations using communication aids usually take place.

There are many differences in conversations between people who speak naturally and those where one individual (or, on rare occasions, both) uses a communication aid. There are great differences between users and the type of aid, but one thing they have in common is that articulation in aided communication differs from and takes longer than that of normal speech, and that the conversational partner has other functions in addition to the usual ones (cf. Kraat, 1985).

Articulation

People who speak naturally do not normally think about how they should pronounce the words they are speaking. They do not think about how they move their tongue or mouth, or how they make their vocal chords vibrate. Apart from those occasions when one is using an unfamiliar word or speaking a foreign language, pronunciation is an automatic process. Only occasionally does one stop and search for the word that best expresses what one wishes to say.

Operating a communication aid is the functional equivalent of pronouncing sounds, but for the individual using a communication aid, the physical formulation is not normally an automatic process. The activity occurs consciously, and takes a considerable portion of the attention and effort that is used to formulate what is to be said. Reduced motor control and involuntary movements can easily lead to the user making mistakes. Imprecise movements may make understanding difficult for the listener if the letter, word or sign is not written on a screen or spoken synthetically. The result may be misunderstandings, a breakdown in communication and frustration. In addition, attention is detracted from what is actually being said.

Time

The time spent pronouncing what is being said is probably the most important difference between natural and aided communication. Even if a speedy communication aid is used, the number of words spoken per minute will be considerably lower than that of natural speech. The low speed means that it takes longer to say what one wants to say, places other demands on the listener (see below), and that the user is unable to take part in so many communicative situations.

The total amount of language spoken by users of communication aids during the course of one day will be considerably lower than that spoken by unaided speakers. Beukelman, Yorkston, Poblete and Naranjo (1984) examined the number of words four adult communication aid users spoke during a period of two weeks. They found that the average number of words spoken during the course of one day varied between 269 and 728 words. This is in stark contrast to the usual number of words spoken by people who do not use communication aids. For example, children between 3 and 12 years of age speak 20–30 000 words a day (Wagner, 1985).

The following example gives a good impression of the time taken for a simple and successful conversation between an aided speaker (A) who points at a board containing letters and a natural speaker (N).

A: (Looks at N to attract his attention and points) *A*
N: (Repeats the letter) *A*
A: (Points at 'space')
N: *A*
A: (Points at letter) *N*
N: *N*

A: (Points at letter) *E*
A: (Points at letter) *E*
N: *N*
A: (Points at letter) *E*
N: *E* (Guesses the word) *NEW*
A: (Points at letter) *W*
N:*W*
A: (Points at letter) *A*
N:*A*
A: (Points at letter) *L*
N:*L*
A: (Points at letter) *L*
N: (Asks) *Do you want one or two L's?*
A: (Points at number) *2*
N: (Guesses) *Oh, did you get a new wallet for Christmas?*
A: (Nods his head) 'Yes'

It took the aided user almost one minute to say what he wanted. After 19 conversational turns the conversational partner (N) has yet to say anything of his own: he has merely interpreted what the user (A) had said. In a conversation between two natural speakers only one of them would have spoken and the sentence, '*I got a new wallet for Christmas*' would have taken 2–3 seconds.

The role of the conversational partner

In ordinary conversations the conversational partners are equal. Both can formulate what they wish to say, and they are not usually dependent on help from the other person in order to express themselves. Users of communication aids experience a totally different situation. The natural speaker must often formulate the user's remarks in addition to his or her own. This is especially true when using graphic signs and limited vocabularies, where the listener has to interpret what the user is trying to say. This takes so long that it may prompt the listener to guess in order to save time, so that it is unnecessary for the user to spell out the whole word. In the example above, the guesswork was beneficial. The user said what he wanted to say quicker than if he had spelled out the whole sentence. However, if the listener guesses wrongly, the remark may take more time instead of less.

In the following example the aided speaker (A) has 50 words on a board and can make a few gestures. The conversational partner (N) is a male nurse (Kraat, 1985).

A: (Points at the communication board) *HOME*
N: *Home? What about home? Is it something to do with your sister?*
A: (Gestures) 'No'
A: (Points at board) *DAYS OF THE WEEK*

N: *Sunday? Monday? Tuesday?...Saturday?*
A: (Gestures) 'Yes'
N: *Something to do with home and Saturday?*
A: (Points at board) *MAN*
N: *A man? Is there a special man who's coming?*
A: (Gestures) 'No'
N: *Shall I find out who the man is?*
A: (Gestures emphatically) 'Yes'
N: *A relative? A friend? Someone at the hospital?*
A: (Gestures) 'Yes'
N: *Someone at the hospital. Let me see, a doctor, therapist, friend?*
N: *Can you give me some more clues?*
A: (Points with his eyes to the top of N's head)
N: *Head. Part of the head. Brain. Does he work with his head?*
A: (Points at board) *COLOUR*

This 'conversation' consisted of over 100 exchanges and lasted for 20 minutes before the nurse understood what the user wanted to ask: *Can Karl* (who was a black guard) *drive me home on Saturday in the hospital van?* It seems correct to say that what the aided speaker wanted to say came out as the result of cooperative effort between the user and the conversational partner. The conversational partner may thus be an important factor in how well an aided speaker can express himself.

Chapter 4
Children and adults in need of augmentative communication

There are a large number of people in need of augmentative communication. Even if one only includes individuals with developmental problems – with whom this book is primarily concerned – the number of people in the United States who are unable to speak is estimated to be around 900 000 (Blackstone and Painter, 1985). There are approximately 240 million inhabitants in the United States compared to 60 million in the United Kingdom, which would suggest that there are approximately 225 000 people of all ages in the UK who are without functional speech as a result of developmental disorders.

In a survey carried out in Washington State in the United States, Matas, Mathy-Laikko, Beukelman and Legresley (1985) discovered that 0.3–0.6 per cent of children of school age were unable to produce speech that was sufficiently understandable for them to use it as their main form of communication. These accounted for 3.5–6 per cent of the children who were given special education. This figure does not take into account children with less extensive speech disorders. If it is assumed that 0.5 per cent of British children between the ages of 1 and 19 are unable to produce sufficiently comprehensible speech for it to serve as their main form of communication, this amounts to 75 000 children and adolescents.

Three functional groups

Individuals who need augmentative communication fall into three main groups, depending on the function the augmentative communication will fill, i.e. the extent to which they need a means of expression, a supportive language or an alternative language. All the three groups are characterised by either not having begun speaking at the usual time or having lost their speech skills as the result of an injury. This makes it difficult for them to communicate with other people. The biggest differences between the groups, and the basis for distinguishing between them, are the varying degrees of language comprehension they display and their ability to learn to understand and use language in the future.

Expressive language group

Children and adults who belong to the expressive language group have a fairly good understanding of other people's speech but are unable to express themselves with the aid of language. The cause of the speech disorder is often a motor handicap, and in the vast majority of cases this is due to brain damage. The purpose of teaching this group an alternative communication form is to provide them with a means of expression that they will be able to use with their reduced motor skills . However, there are also children with normal motor skills who are unable to speak as a result of, for example, a larynx operation (laryngotomy).

For many individuals who belong to the expressive language group, their alternative form of communication will become a *permanent* means of expression – a means of communication the individual will use for the rest of his or her life.

Supportive language group

The supportive language group may be divided into two sub-groups. For the first sub-group, training in an alternative form of communication is for the most part a step toward the development of speech. The augmentative communication is not intended to be a replacement for speech – neither for the individuals concerned nor for those who communicate with them. Its chief function is to encourage the comprehension and expressive use of speech. The most obvious use of augmentative communication as a supportive language is with children whom it is expected will begin to speak but whose language development is very delayed. Children with developmental dysphasia belong to this group, as do many children with Down's syndrome.

The other sub-group of is composed of children and adults who have learned to speak but who have difficulty in making themselves understood. Individuals in this group may need to produce manual signs or point at letters corresponding to the sounds that the listener has not understood. This sub-group of the supportive language group resembles the expressive language group most, but individuals belonging to it do not have augmentative communication as their main form of communication. People with severe articulation disorders may belong to this group.

Using augmentative communication as a supportive language with which to accelerate the use and understanding of speech is easiest when the individual has been diagnosed, if one has a good grasp of how speech usually develops among children with this diagnosis. In the majority of instances, however, conditions initially will not be so clear. This is especially true of children with Down's syndrome. This group includes both children who develop very good speech and children who develop speech that is difficult to understand. One may hope or even believe that a child will learn to speak, but only time will show whether this will be the case.

The incidence of social and mental problems is far greater among children with language disorders than among children in general (Baker and Cantwell, 1982; Ingram, 1959). Language disorders often cause conflicts in the family, and the difficulties and frustration produced may create an exceptionally difficult family situation. One should therefore aim at providing the children in the supportive language group a temporary linguistic instrument that may reduce the negative effects produced by language disorders.

Alternative language group

For individuals who belong to the alternative language group, augmentative communication is the language they will use for the rest of their lives. Augmentative communication is also the language that other people will generally use to communicate with them. This group is characterised by using little or no speech as a means of communication. The aim is therefore that they will use an alternative form of communication as their native language.

Autistic and severely mentally handicapped individuals, among others, belong to the alternative language group. In this group one also finds individuals with *auditive agnosia* or 'language deafness'. The diagnosis of auditive agnosia encompasses children or adults who appear to have special problems in interpreting sounds as meaningful linguistic elements. They have normal hearing in the sense that they can signal that they have registered a sound, but are unable to distinguish between speech sounds and, in severe cases, between, say, a child crying and a foghorn (Arnold, 1965).

Distinguishing between the groups

The purpose of distinguishing between expressive, supportive and alternative language groups is to bring out the fact that there are different objectives for implementing augmentative communication training and that the teaching will differ in each of the groups. Objectives should be formulated on the basis of each individual, and the division into groups may be helpful when formulating these objectives.

The division into three groups does not imply that it is always easy to determine in which group a given individual belongs. It is particularly difficult to distinguish between people who belong to the supportive language group and the alternative language group. This is well illustrated by the experience gained from teaching signs to mentally handicapped and autistic people in recent years. Success has been achieved in teaching signs to people of 40–50 years, who had not learned to speak despite years of speech training, but who have consequently begun to speak. For some of these people, speech has gradually become their main form of communication. Before this it was reasonable to assume that they were incapable of learning to speak.

The most common groups in need of augmentative communication

Among individuals belonging to these three language groups, one finds different clinical groups, and the same clinical groups can be represented in more than one of the three language groups. Some individuals with cerebral palsy need a communication aid in order to be able to express themselves at all; others need a support for speech that is difficult to understand, or may only require an aid for a short period of time. Some autistic people begin speaking after having used signs. Others never learn to understand or use speech but are able to understand and use some manual or graphic signs.

Motor handicap

It is first and foremost children and adults with cerebral palsy who have motor disorders rendering them unable to use speech to communicate. This group includes people who have insufficient control of the speech organs (tongue, mouth, throat, etc.) to be able to articulate language sounds normally (anarthria, dysarthria). They may be paralysed or have spasms that make it difficult for them to control their articulation properly, which makes it difficult for people who do not know them well to understand what they are saying (Hardy, 1983).

Motor disorders that affect only speech are rare. The vast majority of people who have a motor handicap leading to speech loss have also lost other motor functions. They may experience varying degrees of reduced coordination of the hand and finger movements. Many are dependent on wheelchairs or crutches.

Approximately 1 in 1000 children between the ages of 4

and 16 have combined language and motor disorders (Lagergren, 1981). The incidence increases in adolescence, mainly due to traffic injuries and other accidents that cause brain damage. Around half of these children have no functional speech and are totally dependent on a communication aid. Motor handicapped children with some functional speech may also have a need for permanent or temporary aids as supportive forms of communication.

In the United Kingdom, where 700–900 000 children are born every year, 500–600 of them will be born with a motor handicap and will need augmentative communication. The type and extent of the motor handicaps the children suffer from have a direct effect on which form of communication they will be able to utilise. In the majority of cases some type of aid will be required.

For children who grow up with motor disorders, the difficulties they experience in moving and speaking and the influence from their environment both contribute to their development of a passive style. These children often place great demands on their parents. Training, feeding and washing take up a lot of time, and there are few activities that the children and their parents can take part in together. Even when the children are small, their parents consider them to be happiest when they are passive. 'She's as quiet as an angel', and, 'She is so good', are typical remarks made by mothers about their small children with cerebral palsy (Shere and Kastenbaum, 1966).

Smiles, crying and vocalisation are cues for adults' reactions to children, and they play an important role in early interaction. Children with motor handicaps may not be able to smile or vocalise, and their crying may be deviant compared to that of other children. Signals produced by these children are therefore unclear and fairly inconsistent, and it is easy for their parents to misunderstand them. The same applies to their movements. The childrens' reflexes and involuntary movements may affect their attempts to react to both people and events that occur in their environment (Morris, 1981). For example, the sideways movement of the head that is associated with the tonic neck reflex may make adults construe the child's interest in, and attempts at, investigation as a lack of interest or rejection of a person or object (Bottorf and DePape, 1982). These children are often regarded as more alert and interested when they are tense than when their muscle tonus is low (Burkhart, 1987). High muscle tonus leads to reduced motor control and makes interaction more difficult.

Even crying can be less functional among children with motor handicaps than among other children. Parents usually react to their child's crying and interpret it as an expression for different needs, depending on such circumstances as how long it is since the child ate, had its nappy changed, etc. Among children with motor disorders, crying is often caused by matters beyond the parents' control, for example, muscular pains due to increased muscular tension, or pains in internal organs due to curvature of the spine. It may be difficult or impossible to calm the child down, and the parents may become frustrated and feel inadequate. Long-term and frequent bouts of crying can be a source of constant irritation for the parents. If all this is taken into consideration, it is hardly surprising that the parents feel that their children are happy when they are passive.

Over-interpretation, i.e. a tendency on the part of the caregiver to act as though a child is communicating something specific before it is reasonable to assume that the child is really communicating, may be an important force in the child's development (Ryan, 1974; Lock, 1980). When caregivers react to the children's activities in this way, they create conditions in which the child will learn to communicate. Over-interpretation is dependent, however, on the child acting in a manner that the parents can construe as communicative. Children who display few such 'legible' activities (Martinsen, 1980), and this includes children with motor disorders, will often have a poorer language environment, i.e. an environment that shows less reaction to them than it would to normally developed children (Ryan, 1977). Language comprehension may also be reduced, even though the neurological basis for language acquisition has not been affected. Children with extensive motor disorders will lose a significant part of the natural language teaching that other children have. Children in the pre-lingual period cry, laugh, take hold of and reach out for objects, make gurgling noises that may resemble words, etc. These are activities that make parents and other adults react and speak to the children, which indirectly leads to language learning. After the children have begun to speak, they develop their language in a similar way by taking part in conversations. They receive comments about what they themselves say and do, and answers to questions about objects and activities they are interested in or wonder about. Children with motor disorders lose out on many of these experiences, and this may lead to reduced language comprehension and less knowledge about the environment.

The children's physical disabilities place considerable restrictions on their personal development. There are activities in which they will be unable to participate, and many fields where they will gain only limited experience. Part of this limitation is caused primarily not by the motor handicap, however, but by the fact that, due to negative experiences, they believe they are unable to do anything. Later on they will no longer try to do things that they perhaps would have been capable of. They learn that they are dependent on others because others do things for them which they would be unable to manage alone. At the same time they will experience that they are an inconvenience, that they are a hindrance and that the adults are most content when they are passive. The adults' attitude to the children, which the children to a great extent assume themselves (cf. Madge and Fassam, 1982), therefore plays a significant role in forming their life and opportunities for personal growth.

A passive communicative style becomes a general characteristic as the children grow older, and there is reason to believe that the foundation of this is laid already at an early stage. Many children with motor disorders who have experienced affirmation and denial as their only form of communication – a kind of 'Twenty Questions' with, say, eyes up for 'Yes' and down for 'No' – have been given new opportunities with the advent of the new generation of communication aids. However, it appears that they do not initiate conversations, even though they have mastered their communication aid and are able to answer all sorts of questions, not even when it appears as though they have something to say. For children who have grown up with answers to questions as their only communicative strategy, it is difficult to learn to use language in new ways. It is therefore important to find communicative expressions that the children can utilise in order to take the initiative, so that they do not learn that they must wait until others have asked them a question before they say anything.

The level of language comprehension varies considerably among children and adults with speech problems due to motor disorders. Many of the people in this group have normal language comprehension, but a number of them are multi-handicapped and have language disorders resulting from brain damage. For some, augmentative communication will be the form of communication that they understand best. Thus, among those with motor disorders, there will also be people who belong to what we have called the supportive language group and the alternative language group.

Developmental language disorders

In general, children speak their first words between the age of 10 and 13 months, and on average they will begin using two-word sentences by the time they reach 18 months. Approximately 3 per cent of all children have not begun to speak by the time they have reached 2 years, and 4 per cent have not said three words with coherent meaning by the time they have reached 3 years of age (Fundudis, Kolvin and Garside, 1979). The incidence of a serious degree of developmental language disorders is 7–8 in 10 000 (Ingram, 1975).

Children who are considerably more retarded in their language development than in other areas are usually regarded as having specific language disorders. In reality this means the majority of those who are given this diagnosis score within the normal range on a non-verbal intelligence test.

The group is multifarious and contains many variations in terms of special characteristics and the degree of problems. Different sub-groups may be identified on the basis of the scores they achieve in the various types of tasks in the most commonly used intelligence tests, for example, Wechsler Intelligence Scales for Children (WISC). There are also sub-groups that are characterised by different background factors, i.e. they have different histories of development and different forms of associated disorders (Benton, 1977; Cooper and Griffiths, 1977).

Children with developmental language disorders, regardless of which sub-group they belong to, will gradually begin to speak, even though their speech will generally be poorly articulated throughout the pre-school period. This makes these children difficult to understand, although their parents often understand them better than other people can. When the children reach school age, most will have begun to speak clearly enough for even those who do not know them to understand. The retarded language development will, however, mean that the children have a smaller vocabulary, and often less knowledge of their environment, than their peers. The extent to which this happens will vary according to the child's functional level in other areas. Reduced knowledge is characteristic of most children with moderate or more serious developmental language disorders, and will remain so at least until they are well into their school years.

An important sub-group appears to be children with *dyspractic traits*, i.e. children who have difficulty in performing voluntary acts, especially those that require coordinated movement. These children have problems in carrying out practical acts in a large variety of activities, though not to the same extreme degree as girls with Rett's syndrome (see below).

Another important sub-group of children with developmental language disorders are children with the so-called *language disorder syndrome* or 'cluttering' (Arnold, 1965; Weis, 1967). The language disorder syndrome appears to be a genetic speech disorder occurring relatively frequently in families. It is characterised by several successive language disorders; it begins with a delayed onset of speech, followed by difficulty in articulating words and problems with syntax and inflections. In addition, the children show difficulty in perceiving and discriminating between language sounds, clumsiness in carrying out complex movements, and amusicality. The problems of articulation consist in the rate of speech increasing at the end of the word or utterance, and consonantal sounds being pronounced 'carelessly', as though there was a stone in the child's mouth. This poor articulation means that in the first years after learning to speak it is difficult for people other than those who know the child well to understand what is being said. The problems are especially evident when the child becomes excited. Most of these children will speak clearly and be understood by the time they begin at school, except on occasions when they are especially excited. The problems with syntax appear when the children omit words or change their order in a sentence. If they receive only normal reading teaching, they will often develop reading and writing difficulties.

In conversations with other children or adults, children with language disorder syndrome and other children with developmental language disorders will experience that they are not making themselves understood. The difficulties will lead to them getting such meaningless answers as *yes, no,* or *hmm* in response to their communicative efforts no matter what they say, and they will not receive an answer to their questions (Schjølberg, 1984). Adults often solve the problem of not being able to understand by taking control of the interaction with the child: they give more commands and ask fewer questions (Bondurat, Romeo and Kretschmer, 1983). This reduces the pressure on the adult to understand what the child is saying, and at the same time deprives the child of the chance of controlling the interaction on the basis of his or her own interests. In addition to the fact that the children will lose out on this pleasant form of interaction enjoyed by other children, their articulatory disorders also lead to reduced participation in ordinary social interactions. These interactions are a natural form of learning for children and important for the acquisition of language, concepts and knowledge about society.

The problems that adults and other children encounter when with children with language disorders may lead to the children withdrawing from the interaction. Many preschool children with developmental language disorders are shy and timid in the company of others, both among adults whom they do not know and among other children. When they commence school, they often have problems getting along with other children. In extreme cases this may lead to selective mutism, i.e. the children do not speak outside their home, even after they have begun to speak clearly. Others may be naughty and aggressive (Baker and Cantwell, 1982; Ingram, 1959).

It is likely that these childrens' problems are a direct result of the difficulties they experience in making themselves understood. Most social situations require speech. When they meet new people the children are asked such questions as *What is your name?* and *How old are you?*, and must thus reveal their impaired language skills. In some cases children with poor articulation find speaking 'clearly' and understandably to be such a strain that it also becomes more difficult for them to do other things. The specific speech disorder may then spread and become a more extensive problem; a kind of acquired dyspraxia.

Children with developmental language disorders are not taught a form of alternative communication as a means of providing them with a native language. They belong to the *supportive language group*, and are clear examples that augmentative communication is a support in the development of speech. It is most common to use manual signs but other forms of communication have also been used (Hughes, 1974, 1975). Relatively little systematic research has been carried out into the use of sign language in this group, but a good deal of positive clinical experience has been gained. Good results from specific cases have also been reported (Caparulo and Cohen, 1977; von Tetzchner, 1984a).

The effect the signs may have on the children's conversational partners is almost as important as the effect of learning on the children. It can be easy for adults to either overestimate or underestimate how much the children understand. If the children use signs at the same time as they speak, it is easier for the adults to understand and reply to what the children are saying in a meaningful way. For the children this means that the interaction with adults may be more meaningful and pleasurable. At the same time it will be easier for the adults to comment on what the children are doing and tell them about objects and activities that are happening, in the same way as they do when they are with other children. This makes it easier for the children to learn the names of objects, how events are discussed, how objects are used, social rules, etc. If the sign teaching is successful, then one indirect consequence of the sign training may be that the children are less likely to have a poor vocabulary and are more likely to be able to develop concepts.

A third aim of sign teaching, which also builds on indirect effects, is to increase the children's social control. Even after they have begun to speak clearly and make themselves understood, there will be many rules regarding interaction that these children have not learned, but with which their peers are familiar. Improving the children's ability to make themselves understood and increasing their participation in good social interaction may make them less shy and timid,

and will thus help them to enjoy improved social intercourse with their peers and with adults whom they do not
know well.

Mental handicap

Mental handicap is not a professional diagnosis, but rather
an *administrative* category. Traditionally, the term covered
all children who, it was felt, were unable to benefit from
normal schooling, and who ought therefore to attend special schools. Today '...mental handicap is used as a collective term for a whole range of different conditions with
wholly different causes. Common to these, however, is the
fact that the learning ability of those concerned, and their
chances of coping in society, are more or less restricted and
that the condition is visible at an early stage'
(Lossiusutvalget [The Lossius Committee], 1985).

There are a number of sub-groups of mental handicap.
In some instances the reason for the mental handicap is
known, but in approximately half the cases the cause is
unknown (Kirman, 1985). The largest single group are
people with Down's syndrome, who account for approximately 20 per cent of those with mental handicap.

It is usual to distinguish between the different degrees
of mental handicap on the basis of scores in intelligence
tests. An intelligence quotient (IQ) between 69 and 55 is
considered a mild degree, an IQ between 54 and 40 as a
moderate degree, an IQ between 39 and 25 a severe degree
and an IQ below 24 a profound degree of mental handicap.
However, it is essential to remember that an IQ does not
say much about an individual. The group of mentally handicapped people contains wholly different individuals with
very different developmental backgrounds. The score
attained on the intelligence test conceals these differences
to a far greater extent than it reveals them. Even what we
may call the ability to learn varies considerably among
people with the 'same' level of intelligence. It is especially
difficult to predict linguistic skills on the basis of the score
attained on an IQ test. For people who achieve a score of
more than 40–50, there is no connection between IQ and
the milestones in language development, i.e. the time at
which individuals begin to speak and they time they produce their first word combinations. Among people who
achieve an IQ score lower than 40–50, it is difficult both
practically and theoretically to distinguish between poor
language and communicative ability and other cognitive
functions. Performance on intelligence tests is dependent,
among other things, on the fact that the test instructions
have been understood. Among those who have the poorest
linguistic and communicative qualifications, this condition

is difficult to fulfil. Poor linguistic skills also prevent people from learning other skills that are measured in intelligence tests. One therefore finds a clear statistical correlation between the IQ score and linguistic skills among people with moderate and severe degrees of mental handicap. But even though a smaller proportion of low-functioning mentally handicapped individuals develop language than those who function rather better, one may also find instances of individuals from the weakest group developing language.

Among people with mental handicap, there is a high frequency of multiple handicap. At a large Norwegian institution 30 per cent of the inhabitants had non-correctable visual impairments. Of these, 7 per cent were totally blind and 11–12 per cent were functionally blind, i.e. there was nothing wrong with the eye itself, but rather with the regions of the brain concerned with visual perception (S. Spetalen, personal communication, 1990). In addition, even minor visual problems have greater consequences for mentally handicapped people than for others. Among those who are most seriously mental handicapped, compensating for loss of sight is often problematic because spectacles are easily broken and contact lenses may cause injury. Hearing impairments are also more frequent among mentally handicapped people. For example, in an English survey 8 per cent of mentally handicapped children in institutions were found to be deaf. In the same survey 14 per cent were found to be so physically handicapped that they were unable to move on their own (Kirman, 1985).

Owing to the great differences in functional levels and the high incidence of sensory loss and motor handicaps, all forms of augmentative communication may be of interest for the mentally handicapped group. Some will belong to the expressive language group, others to the supportive or alternative language group.

Children with Down's syndrome constitute the largest and best-documented single group (cf. Gibson, 1978; Nadel, 1988) and will therefore be used to illustrate the collective category 'mental handicap'. However, it is important to stress the great differences one finds both between and within the individual sub-groups.

Children with Down's syndrome often have a need for a supportive language, even though a number also belong to the alternative language group. Smith and von Tetzchner (1986) investigated 10 3-year-olds with Down's syndrome. On the basis of the information given by the children's parents, it was found that the children used an average of 45 words. The number of words used by each child varied between 0 and 250. At the age of 5, only one of the children had a mean length of utterance of more than 1.5 words, implying that most of the utterances produced by

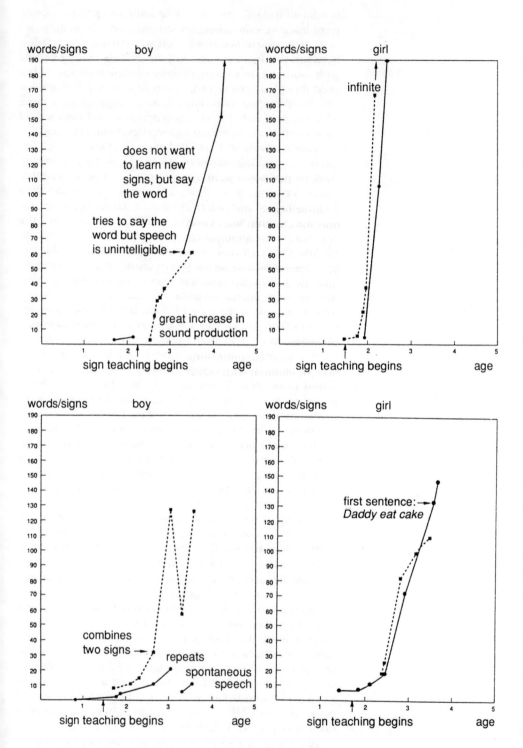

Figure 23. *Sign development among four children with Down's syndrome.*

■ manual signs
● spoken words

the other children were one-word utterances.

Compared with normally developed children, children with Down's syndrome have a significantly delayed language development. How quickly children with Down's syndrome acquire speech is related to their development in other areas, and the extent to which they are able, or permitted, to interact with their caregivers. The children's participation in social interaction with others, and thus their opportunities for natural, indirect language and concept learning, is affected by the fact that they spend more time processing and reacting to impressions than other children, and that they often have such a low level of activity that the interaction is controlled by adults (cf. Ryan, 1977).

In principle, the objective of augmentative communication for children with Down's syndrome is – as with children with developmental language disorders – to accelerate the acquisition of speech and increase the quality of interaction in the period before they begin to speak. At the same time an alternative language will be secured for the few who develop little or no speech. The similarity to children with developmental language disorders is emphasised by the fact that children with Down's syndrome often have pronunciation that can be very difficult to understand.

The most common form of augmentative communication for children with Down's syndrome is manual signs. In recent years training of this type has been carried out in several countries, and the great majority of reports have been positive (Johansson, 1987; Prevost, 1983). In the county of North Trøndelag in Norway, the experiences gained from using manual signs among eight mentally handicapped children were systematically registered (Rostad, 1989). Four of these children have Down's syndrome. It was noted how old each child was when the training was started, at the acquisition of each new sign, how old the children were when they began to speak, and when each new word was first spoken.

The four children with Down's syndrome learned both manual signs and spoken words during the course of the training (Figure 23). All of them learned signs first. The acquisition of manual signs and spoken words was slow to begin with but gradually became more rapid. Progress was noted first in the use of signs. Gradually the children began to learn more words than signs, and the number of signs they learned levelled off and decreased. This regularity in the increase of words in relation to the use of manual signs, together with the fairly large age difference in terms of when the sign training began, suggests that the training had a positive – perhaps directly catalytic – effect on the development of speech.

It must be stressed, however, that teaching the use of

manual signs did not have the same effect on all the mentally handicapped children in the survey. For one of the four children who did not have Down's syndrome, the development took a different course. This child did not benefit from the sign teaching, but gradually learned to say many words. This highlights the fact that there is no single form of augmentative communication that suits everyone.

Autism

In most cases the onset of the autistic syndrome occurs before the age of 2. The description of the disorder varies according to age. The three main characteristics of autism are *extensive language and communication disorders, difficulty in relating to others* and *abnormal reactions to the environment*.

The incidence of autism varies somewhat according to how strictly the diagnostic criteria are interpreted. If the classic criteria are taken strictly, then the incidence is 1 in 10 000. On the basis of the most common interpretation of the criteria, the incidence is approximately 2–4 in 10 000. In Norway it is reckoned that the incidence of autism is 5–6 in 10 000. Use of the new DSM-III-R criteria will increase the incidence somewhat (Table 2). At least twice as many boys as girls have autism. The causes of the syndrome are not known but there are clear indications that the difficulties have a biological basis. It is believed that the condition has several causes.

Almost 50 per cent of autistic adults have no functional speech (Rutter, 1985). Among those who learn to speak, linguistic development is often delayed and language skills extremely varied. Some autistic people use neither signs nor speech and have almost no understanding of language. Others can speak and understand a lot. Still others gradually build up a large vocabulary, use seemingly normal syntax and are able to express thoughts, feelings and needs. The vast majority of those who do begin to speak display to begin with a high degree of echolalia, i.e. the reiteration of words and phrases out of context. They rarely initiate contact with other people. Even those autistic people who function best often speak in 'monologues', i.e. without taking heed of the listener, and they often take what other people have said quite literally.

There are also great differences in terms of non-verbal skills. Some autistic people have an even skill profile, while others are more skilled in some areas than in others. In surveys where large groups of autistic children and adolescents have been followed up into adulthood, it appears that there is a relationship between the functional level and the extent to which the autistic individual began to use language in the

Table 2. *Diagnostic criteria from DSM-III-R, the revised edition of DSM-III. At least 8 of the 16 criteria listed in the table must be apparent, including at least two from A, one from B and one from C. NB: Criteria are said to exist only if behaviour is deviant in relation to the individual's developmental level.*

A. Qualitative deficits in social interaction with others. Apparent in:

1. Pervasive lack of understanding of the fact that other people exist, or that other people have feelings.
2. Seeks comfort in deviant ways.
3. Deficient imitation of others.
4. Lack of or deviant social play.
5. Severely impaired ability to get along with peers.

B. Qualitative deficits in verbal and non-verbal communication, and in activities requiring imagination. Apparent in:

1. No form of communication such as gurgling noises, facial expressions, use of gestures or speech.
2. Pervasive deviant non-verbal communication such as eye contact, facial expression, posture or use of gestures in order to initiate or influence social interaction.
3. Lack of activities that require imagination.
4. Pervasive deviant speech, including volume, vocal.register, accentuation, tempo, rhythm and intonation.
5. Pervasive deviation in the form or content of speech, including stereotypical and repetitive speech.
6. Pervasive impaired ability to initiate and carry on a conversation with other people, despite the fact that the speech of the individual is in all other respects adequate.

C. Severely limited behavioural repertoire and few interests. Apparent in:

1. Stereotypical activities such as flipping with the hands, twirling things, banging the head and complex body movements (rocking, etc.).
2. Persistent preoccupation with objects or dependence on unusual objects.
3. Pervasive negative reactions to change in trivial aspects of the environment.
4. Unreasonable demands to follow routines to the very last detail.
5. Limited interests, and a preoccupation with special interests.

D. Onset during the infant years

pre-school period. The degree of meaningful speech that occurs before an autistic individual has reached the age of 6 has proved to be the best indicator of later functional levels, both linguistic and non-linguistic. In a Norwegian survey of 64 autistic children and adolescents, little progress was evident in the quality of language from pre-school age to early adulthood (A.M. Kvale, H. Martinsen and S. Schjølberg, unpublished data). The few exceptions to this rule were among children who had been given systematic sign teaching.

The unusual reactions to other people are closely linked to the extensive communicative and language problems experienced by autistic people. Autistic babies and infants have fewer of the normal behavioural forms on which early communication between children and adults is based, and their parents feel that it is difficult for them to achieve contact with their child. The children seem uninterested, do not appear to react when they are being played with or tended to, do not like to cuddle, are difficult to calm down when they cry, and often appear content when left alone. In infancy they often dislike being lifted up, and do not usually mould their bodies to the body of the person who is carrying them, as children normally do. Many autistic people like bodily contact, while others shriek, become tense and seem afraid when they are touched. Eye contact is often missing. Some autistic people merely cast a fleeting glance at the face of the person with whom they are interacting, others stare and scrutinise the face at close quarters. When in groups with other children or adolescents, they appear to show little interest in what the others are doing, and seldom learn by imitating others.

'Unusual reactions to the surroundings' includes a long list of peculiarities that occur in varying degrees within the group. Among those characteristics that are most commonly mentioned are negative reactions to the fact that fixed routines are broken and that surroundings change. Many autistic people react to changes with displays of anger or fear.

Most autistic people are only rarely self-occupied. They have a limited range of activities, and can carry on performing those same activities for long periods of the day over months and years. 'Unusual reactions to their surroundings' is also an expression of the fact that autistic children are generally interested in different activities from most children. In particular, many of them are interested in objects that revolve or can be twirled, and in flashing lights. Normal toys are usually of no interest. Typical examples of favourite activities are wandering aimlessly, twirling and spinning things round like a whirligig, filling a basin with water, leafing through books, turning lights on and off, tapping objects and listening to music. Closely linked to this are the stereotyped acts which characterise the group. These include sitting and rocking, 'flipping' with their fingers or objects they are holding, 'filtering' light through the fingers, twining hair, waving arms, banging the head against objects and twisting the body, arms or hands into unusual positions.

Many autistic people react abnormally to external stimuli. Some autistic children do not seem to react to voices, and may be suspected of deafness. Even among well-functioning autistic children and adults, it can be difficult to know whether they are listening when being spoken to and interested in what is being said. Some autistic people are oversensitive to sounds. Normal sounds are troublesome and sometimes painful, especially in periods where the autistic individual is under a lot of pressure. Some autistic individuals have no visible reaction to pain, which has led to speculation that they have a reduced sense of pain. Other autistic children are oversensitive to touch (Grandin, 1989). Children who early in life show no signs of feeling pain, however, do show this when their general functional level improves. Many autistic children and adults also react abnormally to visual stimuli. With the exception of autistic people who also have visual defects or reduced sight or hearing, however, no specific sensory deviations have been found. The deviations seem rather to be linked to perceptual processing (Hermelin and O'Connor, 1970).

Considering the relatively poor prognosis autistic children have in terms of developing language, it is natural to give them training in augmentative communication. Since it is assumed from the outset that over 50 per cent of autistic children will never begin to speak and additionally lack language comprehension, it is fair to assume that augmentative communication will often become their main form of communication, an alternative native language. On the basis of their abilities, many autistic children will therefore belong to the alternative language group, but for a large proportion of autistic individuals the augmentative communication will be a supportive language.

Autistic people can utilise different forms of augmentative communication. Manual signs, different graphic systems, script and pictures have all been used. However, manual signs are the most common (cf. Kiernan et al., 1982). In Norway, for example, the majority of autistic children who have not learned to speak receive training in the use of manual signs. In recent years it has become more common to introduce autistic children systematically to manual signs as soon as they have been diagnosed, despite the fact that it is too early to expect these children to have begun to speak.

Experiences from teaching autistic children to use signs are unequivocally positive, and include cases where sign training has been used to improve the speech of those who are able to speak. Not all sign teaching has led to the acquisition of many signs, but almost all the autistic people have at least learned some signs, often in a short space of time. Among autistic individuals who have profited the most from sign teaching, following several years of training, one may find the spontaneous use of long sentences of signs, and – among some exceptional individuals – a sign vocabulary of several hundred signs. It seems realistic to assume that even the least functional autistic individuals will be able to acquire between five and ten signs after approximately two years of training. This may seem like a modest objective, but even such a limited improvement in an autistic individual's capacity for self-expression and understanding of others can have a great significance for everyday well-being, provide an opportunity to learn necessary social and practical skills, and improve the general quality of life.

Autistic people in all age groups are very different from one another, and the diagnosis describes a multifarious group. There is great variation in skills among both children and adults, and even the most striking characteristics of this group – such as the fact that they are preoccupied with special things, react negatively to change, are sensitive to sound, etc. – are not apparent in all autistic individuals. Intervention for autistic people must therefore be individually planned.

Rett's syndrome

Rett's syndrome is a progressive neurological condition that affects girls only. Their development is seemingly normal until the age of 6–18 months, although in retrospect it may appear that they were also more passive than other infants before the disease became apparent. After the age of 6–18 months they begin to lose previously acquired skills. The circumference of the head is normal at birth but growth slows, and the circumference is then less than normal. Epilepsy is common and may appear at any age.

Rett's syndrome has an incidence of 1 in 20000 of the population, i.e. it occurs in 1 in every 10000 girls (Hagberg, 1985). Its aetiology is presently unknown, and there is no medical test that can determine if a girl has the syndrome. The course of development determines the diagnosis, and it can be difficult to give a reliable diagnosis before the girl has reached the age of 3–4 years (Hagberg and Witt-Engerström, 1986).

Rett's syndrome was not considered a syndrome before 1983. Previously the girls were often diagnosed as being autistic. The fact that Rett's syndrome has only recently become known also means that a number of important questions about the functional level of the girls remain unanswered. One of the most important questions is the extent to which there is a correlation between the inability of the girls to express themselves and their ability to understand the speech of others. There are observations that may indicate that at least some of the girls have some understanding of language, despite the fact that they are almost totally incapable of expressing themselves.

Hagberg and Witt-Engerström (1986) have suggested four stages of development in Rett's syndrome (Table 3).

Table 3. *The four clinical stages in the development of Rett's syndrome (from Hagberg and Witt-Engerstrøm, 1986).*

1. The first stage (the early onset stagnation stage) lasts for several months between the ages of approximately 6–18 months. There is decelerating skull growth. Development ceases and eye contact and communication worsens. Interest in play diminishes. There is a certain degree of hand waving.

2. The second stage (the rapid destructive stage) lasts for several weeks between the ages of 1 and 3 or 4 years. Development is characterised by rapid deterioration. The girls appear severely mentally handicapped, with typical hand stereotypies and social withdrawal. There is a gradual loss of hand skill/use, while motor skills such as walking are better preserved. The girls are clumsy, however, and display poor balance when walking and standing. They often breathe erratically, and may hyperventilate and gulp air so that their stomachs become distended. At this age they may also experience epileptic fits.

3. The third stage (the pseudostationary stage) lasts for several years during pre- and early school years. The condition appears more stable. They appear to be severely mentally handicapped, but they no longer appear as autistic. Emotional contact is possible. Motor skills such as those used for walking deteriorate. The girls walk with their legs far apart, unsteadily and unbalanced. Epilepsy is common.

4. The fourth stage (the late motor deterioration stage) may begin when females are 5–10–15–25–? years of age and lasts for many years. They lose the ability to walk and will need a wheelchair. General growth stops and they remain small. Pubescent development is normal. They develop curvature of the spine (scoliosis), and the soles of the feet begin to curve in toward the underside of the feet (trophic feet disturbances). Epilepsy is often less problematic and the emotional contact improves. The gaze is an unfathomable stare.

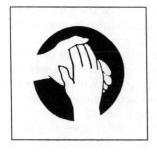

The stages may differ in length, however, and the course of development varies considerably. Not all of the characteristics occur to the same extent among all the girls.

Most of the girls – though not all – develop a special hand stereotypy, in which the hands are rubbed in a sort of 'washing action' which is performed most of the day. Many girls may also sit and open and close their hands almost incessantly. Stereotypical washing actions are fairly common among children with mental handicap or autism, but not to the extent that is typically found among girls with Rett's syndrome. The movements have therefore become a 'trademark' for these patients and appears in the Rett's Syndrome Association logo.

During the course of the disease, hand control deteriorates. Fine motor skills worsen and gradually the girls are no longer able, for example, to use a pincer grip to pick up things. One result of the girls' steadily deteriorating control over their hands is that they lose the ability to play with and manipulate objects. They clutch at things with a 'pawing' movement and grasp objects with their whole hand. It becomes difficult for them to get hold of things, and they drop them easily, so they have increasing problems occupying themselves and doing things on their own initiative, and become more dependent on others.

Perhaps the most characteristic feature of Rett's syndrome is *apraxia*, i.e. the inability to perform voluntary actions. The apraxia is apparent not only in the problems the girls have in learning new skills, but also in the implementation and carrying out of activities that they have already mastered. Even the act of beginning to walk or lifting a leg to walk up a flight of stairs can take a long time, and they may need help in getting started. Another characteristic of apraxia is that it increases with excitement, so that when motivation increases, the action becomes more difficult to perform. It is commonly noted that the girls function best in tranquil surroundings where they are under little pressure. Intervention is therefore aimed at helping them to perform actions, thereby lessening their frustration.

Among girls with Rett's syndrome there is also a strong tendency to hyperventilate. This hyperventilation can be so strong that it leads to fainting. It appears to be related to the fact that the girls become excited; in particular, it often seems to happen when something occurs that they are interested in, or have a strong wish for. It can seem as though they become excited and frustrated over not achieving things, not getting hold of something, being unable to perform actions or express something. It is often in situations of this kind that the hand stereotypies increase, which also happens when the girls are left to manage on their own (Lindberg, 1987). It is therefore important to find a balanced degree of stimulation.

Girls with Rett's syndrome almost never speak, and they are dependent on alternative communication to express themselves. Because of their difficulties in using their hands, manual signs are unsuitable. Aided communication is therefore a natural choice.

However, using communication aids is not easy for them either. Even a simple motor movement such as pointing may be difficult. If their attention is concentrated on the action, in this case the pointing, this may exacerbate the apraxia. Instead attention should be focused on the object at which the girl is pointing.

It is important that communication aids are chosen that can be used even after the loss of motor skills is well advanced. For example, the girls are often able to use simple switches, which do not require fine motor skills, for a long while after they have lost most of the functional motor skills in the hand. Eye pointing seems to be a useful alternative for those girls who are unable to point or whose hands perform stereotypical movements incessantly. However, with eye pointing also, it is important not to focus on the action because there are examples of apraxia appearing in the use of eye pointing. Perhaps the reason that it works so well is precisely because it is not usual to attempt to influence the gaze and drawn the girl's attention to it.

There are no documented examples of girls with Rett's syndrome being taught augmentative communication, and it is our impression that such training has been rare.

It is assumed that the girls' understanding of language is severely limited. However, it is difficult for people with apraxia, and great difficulty in expressing themselves, to show that they understand. There are, though, a number of accounts of the girls laughing at the right moment, showing interest when a person is mentioned, etc.

> A girl with Rett's syndrome was in town with her father. They stood for a long time waiting at a pedestrian crossing for the 'red man' to change to green. Her father talked while the girl stared in fascination at the traffic light. During the evening meal that same evening the girl suddenly said 'Red man' (Lindberg, 1987).

> A girl with Rett's syndrome had her grandfather to stay. When he came down to eat breakfast, she said clearly 'Hi Grandad!' (Lindberg, 1987).

Girls with Rett's syndrome have also reacted positively to the use of digitised speech.

> Dawn is a 7-year-old girl with Rett's syndrome. As part of her

training in augmentative communication, a communication aid with digitised speech, Alltalk, was tried out. Dawn had a picture of a glass of milk and a biscuit on her talking aid. When she pressed the pictures, the machine said, 'chocolate milk' and 'biscuit'. Once she held her hand on the picture of milk while she was drinking and the machine continued saying, 'chocolate milk', 'chocolate milk'. Dawn laughed heartily. Despite the fact that she had only tried Alltalk a few times and it was difficult to press the pictures, Dawn was very interested and appeared very active when she was using it (von Tetzchner and Øien, 1989).

These observations may indicate that the girls have more understanding of language than is generally thought. The limited results obtained from teaching the girls to express themselves seem to suggest that it is scarcely possible to improve their understanding through use of communication aids. This means that, despite their limited understanding of language, they belong to the *expressive language group*.

Some common problems

A number of problems often occur when teaching people with communication disorders. These problems are often related to the fact that learning takes time and can be difficult to transfer to new situations, and that the individual who is learning has become passive or dependent on others.

Learning takes time

One of the most common barriers in language training is that the teaching can be extremely time-consuming. Some people with communication disorders may take years to learn even seemingly simple skills. This applies to a greater extent to some sub-groups of mentally handicapped and autistic children and adolescents, but is also true of some children with developmental language disorders.

Some professionals take the progress or lack of progress shown by the individual as a measure of their own success. They may therefore set themselves unrealistic aims and be impatient about results. This may result in the training ending too early and other teaching methods being tried instead. It is important to assess one's own efforts, but this assumes that the efforts have been tried out long enough and that one has feasible short- and long-term aims.

The protracted teaching time also has other consequences. One indirect consequence is the fact that the people who take the longest time to learn are also those who are most prone to breaks in continuity. They may have to change schools, or new teachers may be recruited who have insufficient knowledge of what they know and can do and are unaware of how the teaching has been organised. Breaks in continuity may lead to established skills not being reacted to, and these may therefore be forgotten or 'unlearned'. New teachers may try to teach individuals something they already know, or teach them new ways of expressing things that they can already express. Discontinuities and changes in learning routines cause frustration and often lead to behavioural problems, which in turn will make the learning situation even worse.

There are examples where years of training for autistic and mentally handicapped people have been rendered worthless as the result of a change in, or the loss of, an educational programme (Kollzinas, 1984). The negative consequences are further reinforced by the fact that there is a great danger that the skills acquired by those people who function lowest will disappear altogether if training is not continued.

Generalisation

A great problem encountered in teaching is that skills learned in a teaching situation are not transferred to other situations. This is a problem that affects a large number of people in need of augmentative communication, not only those who function poorly. Even when special emphasis has been placed on making conditions favourable for transferral of skills, the results have been unsatisfactory. When the problems of transferring knowledge to new situations are seen in relation to the fact that the training takes a long time, it is important that, in so far as it is practical, the teaching of language and communication is located in natural situations where one can be sure that the skills being taught will be useful for the individual. This means that time must be spent assessing the environment and finding situations where communication can be used functionally and that are also suitable for training purposes. If teaching is planned in other situations, it is important that there is also a plan for how the transferral to new situations will take place.

Learned passivity and dependence on others

In early language teaching it is often necessary to help individuals to some degree. Even though this help may be absolutely necessary, it also represents a problem. The individuals often become dependent on the help and will be unable to use their skills spontaneously.

The dependence associated with language learning is related to the great degree of passivity and dependence on others found in all groups in need of augmentative communication. People who belong to the expressive language group share the characteristic that, in the majority of situations and especially with regard to self-expression, they have been dependent on other people helping them. This antecedent creates habits and ways of adapting to communication that may be difficult to alter when one attempts to give them new means of expressing themselves.

People who belong to the supportive or alternative language group may develop a similar dependence on others. It is not uncommon for children with delayed language development to ask their parents to speak for them when strangers approach them, even after their speech is understood by others. In cases where the childrens' mobility is not impaired, the lack of initiative to communicate is most apparent. For example, among autistic children who are unable to speak, the incidence of communicative episodes is extremely low in comparison with other children, and it is particularly communication initiated by the autistic children that is lacking. For these groups too, it is therefore important that the communication does not become responsive, i.e. that the individual answers only when spoken to by others or takes the 'initiative' after they being urged to do so. Even though it is unintentional on the part of the person who plans the training, the teaching may reinforce a child's dependence.

Chapter 5
Assessment

The need for total intervention

The vast majority of children, adolescents and adults in need of augmentative communication also require other forms of intervention. This is increasingly true the more pervasive the disability. Individuals with the most extensive and complex disabilities will require intervention and support throughout their lives. The primary objective should be that the sum of interventions provides the individual with the best quality of life that is possible.

The different forms of intervention are aimed at providing life-qualities that most people take for granted: a place to live, a job – or at least meaningful employment – meaningful leisure time and pleasure in the company of others; family especially, but preferably friends as well. Individuals should also experience control and choice in their own life, and feel a sense of self-respect.

People in need of augmentative communication run the risk of losing all these life-qualities: only when a reasonable form of total intervention exists can these objectives be realised. Viewing the measures as one entity is the best guarantee for the quality of life. Language and communication training that do not take into account the total life situation of the person concerned, and do not contribute to an overall improvement, are inadequate in terms of the individual's interests, and will probably be poor training as well.

The training should form an integral part of the total intervention, i.e. it should be coordinated with other interventionary measures. This applies in particular to teaching of self-help, work activities and activities that lay the foundations for improved social contact with other people. The content of the teaching is chosen on the basis of a comprehensive assessment of what will benefit the individual most.

What should be included in the total intervention, and how each element should be assessed on its own and in relation to the total intervention, will only be outlined here. The various elements that make up a good total intervention must always be adapted to the needs of the individual and will also vary for each of the different groups in need of augmentative communication.

Assessment methods

Tests

Formal tests have varying value in an assessment, depending on the group in question. This applies both to general intelligence tests and to tests directed at more limited fields such as language understanding, drawing skills and motor development. Structured testing may provide information that is useful for determining the form and content of language and communication training, but it is still a good rule to ask how the test results will be utilised before a test is carried out.

A number of conditions limit the use of the ordinary tests among people in need of augmentative communication. Many individuals have disabilities that prevent the tests being administered in the usual way. This is true, for example, of people with extensive comprehension problems, motor disorders, or visual and hearing impairments. Most tests are based on the assumption that individual can see, hear, understand instructions and speak, as well as move building bricks or other objects. Typical test items are answering questions or following instructions, drawing figures, or building patterns with building bricks and repeating sequences of numbers. Many of the tasks must be completed within a time limit.

Few tests are constructed so that they may be taken by people with handicaps. In order to use the tests among these groups, it is necessary to change the instructions, the method of presentation and often what is expected in reply. Completing a test with adapted testing procedures of this kind implies, however, that the test's usual norms cannot be used, and that the result cannot be interpreted in the usual way. The norms are based on the test being completed in the prescribed manner.

It may still be useful to administer tests. They have the advantage that one knows how normal children score on similar tasks, and over time one may gain experience of how a specific group usually accomplishes the tasks.

Age scores and standard scores

If the use of tests is to be beneficial, then the test results must be used in a meaningful way. In many instances the results achieved are 'translated' to an age score. This may be a straightforward way of describing a child's functional level, but it will often give the wrong impression. For example, even though a 20-year-old boy manages to solve the same tasks on a test as an average 3-year-old, he will nonetheless differ considerably from 3-year-olds. It is better to use standard scores, which indicate how the individual accomplishes a given task in relation to other children of the same age. The advantage of standard scores is that they bring out the variations in a specific age group. An age score gives the average of the age level.

Standard scores are based on a distribution curve where the average is 0 and a certain proportion of the scores fall within each standard score (Figure 24). For example, 68 per cent of the scores will be between +1 standard score and –1 standard score, and this is often termed the normal area. However, there has to be a difference of more than two standard scores from the average before one may speak of a significant deviation. In most intelligence tests the standard score is approximately 15 points, so that an IQ score of 70 is two standard scores below 100, which is the average performance of all persons of a given age. An IQ score of 70 is also usually considered the borderline for mental handicap.

There are many examples of how age scores can be misleading. The score on Reynell's language test levels out at the age of 4, so that small raw score differences may give great variations in age scores (see Reynell, 1969). If a 6-year-old obtains a raw score of 13 in the sub-test 'Verbal expression'

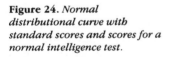

Figure 24. *Normal distributional curve with standard scores and scores for a normal intelligence test.*

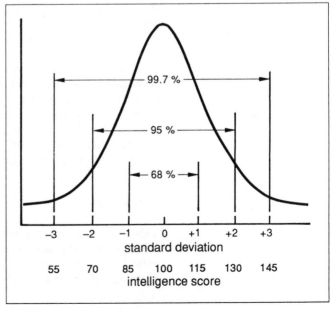

in the Illinois Test of Psycholinguistic Ability (ITPA, Gjessing and Nygaard, 1975), this will give a standard score of −1. This means that the child's skills lie within the normal area, although in the lower region. This sub-test consists, however, of tasks where the frequency of solution changes little with age, and the same raw score is equivalent to the average performance obtained by children of 4;3, which is also the age score. It may be a dramatic experience for the parent of a 6-year-old to learn that he is on the same level as a 4-year-old. It may give a more correct picture of the child's skills to say that he or she is somewhat slow in the ability to express him- or herself, but within what is regarded as normal.

Test profiles

Some tests provide little information about the individual skills in which one is interested when planning intervention for individuals with language disorders. In many intelligence tests most people with poor language skills will obtain poor results, because the tests are designed to distinguish between people who belong to a normal population, not to give information about people with special disabilities. When tests are devised and their scores standardised, individuals in institutions and special schools are not usually included in the sample (cf. Undheim, 1978). Thus, intelligence tests do not discriminate well those who score on the lowest part of the scale.

Most people with poor language skills will achieve irregular test profiles. The tests are designed, however, so that the different sub-tests correlate reasonable well with one another, i.e. an individual will normally perform similarly on the various sub-tests. The irregular profiles found in the efforts of many individuals with language disorders show that the test conditions are not satisfactorily taken into account. It is therefore difficult to predict other skills on the basis of the tests. This is critical in test use, because it is in fact the motivation for devising the tests. Tests are used to gain *general* information about what may be expected of the individuals who are being tested, not to find out how they cope with the random collection of tasks that make up the tests.

Check-lists

A check-list consists of questions about individuals and the environment in which they live. While tests measure an individual's performance in standard situations, check-lists are filled out on the basis of observations or interviews with people who know the individual well. Some check-lists are intended to describe skills (Kiernan and Reid, 1987; Sparrow, Balla and Cicchetti, 1984), others are meant to facilitate diagnosis (Rimland, 1971; Schopler et al., 1980).

It is often practical to use check-lists to assess everyday skills. Check-lists pose questions about different skills on relatively detailed levels, and cover such areas as self-help skills, social skills, behavioural problems and communication. Concrete questions about necessary everyday activities are asked. These include such activities as dressing, eating, going to the toilet, etc. The best check-lists will contain many questions about each particular domain, so that it is possible to draw up profiles. Check-lists often lack questions about the type and amount of help that is required, i.e. how much help the person must have in order to carry out a specific activity and in which situations it is mastered. This is information that will be needed by the person who is planning the intervention.

The Vineland Adaptive Behavior Scale (Sparrow et al., 1984) is often used, and gives a comprehensive representation of the level of skills. A Norwegian check-list has also been developed for use with autistic people and others with similar disorders (Siverts, 1982). This check-list provides an opportunity of describing the type and amount of help that is needed for the individual to be able to carry out specific skills. The problem with this check-list is that it is not standardised, and it is therefore impossible to compare the results obtained with what is normal for the age group in general. For many autistic and mentally handicapped people, the ways in which they differ from their peers are so obvious that the question of how great these differences are is of little significance. The aim is first and foremost to discover which skills the person has, and to build on these in subsequent intervention.

Information from those in contact with the individual

Information from parents and other people who know the individual well is collected through conversations and interviews, and represents in many ways a continuation of the check-lists. However, this information is more detailed and of more direct relevance for the person and his or her environment than similar information obtained from the check-lists, which have standard questions. The information acquired from those in contact with the individual is not only useful in ascertaining the skills he or she possesses, it also provides details about the opinions and views of those in contact with the individual.

Systematic observation

Regardless of the type of disability, systematic observation is always an important part of the assessment. It is important to observe the person in different situations and activities, in the company of others or alone.

Video

In recent years video recordings have played an increasing role in the observation of disabled people. Because they are relatively permanent, video recordings can always be viewed again. Information that crops up at a later stage, or circumstances one did not notice immediately, can be checked. Several people may view a video together and look at specific sequences several times. Video recordings also make it easier to document progress among children who are slow developers.

Video recordings are also a good starting point for discussions with the parents and other people in close contact with an individual. They can say whether the behaviour demonstrated in the video is typical, and can confirm or invalidate assumptions about what the person can and cannot do. By looking at video recordings, innovative ideas for new forms of intervention and communication situations may spring to mind.

Experimental teaching

The first assessment will not always give clear answers to the question of which teaching strategies may be best suited for the individual. Experimental teaching may be required before a decision is made as to how to continue. Such teaching may be regarded as part of the assessment.

Basic information

People in need of augmentative communication are of all ages and have very different skill levels.

To begin with the emphasis should be on the principal issues, to find out what is required in order to get started. Among these issues is the question of the objectives of the language and communication training, i.e. whether the person needs augmentative communication as an expressive means, as a support in order to develop speech, or as an alternative form of language. Even though it is often not possible to answer this question, it helps to focus on what is fundamental to communication teaching. In addition, information is required about such central areas as social functioning, activity level, comprehension of everyday situations, self-help skills, the general level of knowledge and behavioural problems.

Once these steps have been completed the assessment should follow a plan and be be carried out stage by stage. The first step is to outline a plan and the information that forms its basis. The need for more precise information will increase as the problems gradually become clearer. The result of the planned intervention will form a significant part of a continuous assessment.

It is important that the assessment does not delay the implementation of interventionary measures, if there is already sufficient information for these to be effected. Often, intervention is postponed because part of the assessment takes too long. For example, with children with motor disorders, it often seems that the child is assumed to have other disorders, and, for example, language intervention is postponed until the child has demonstrated an understanding of language. The communication aid is thus used to reveal skills instead of contributing to their development.

To begin with it is easy to ask too many questions. This may lead to extra work, and can sometimes make cooperation difficult. In particular, many parents have experienced professionals asking for detailed information that has never been used. Nor is it uncommon for time to be spent carrying out tests and investigations that are never used as the basis for intervention.

Overview of the day

Before beginning with language and communication intervention, it is necessary to have an overview of the activities in which the person already participates. An overview of this kind is the quickest way of gaining insight into the total need for intervention, and gives a suggestion of the individual's strengths and weaknesses. The overview also provides information about what teaching is already taking place. In this way, new interventionary measures can be planned so that they do not disturb current positive activities, and so that they enhance the totality. The overview should include all hours of the day, and be sufficiently detailed that all activities occurring during the course of the day are clearly discernible.

A *day clock* is a useful aid for presenting and structuring the information. A day clock consists of fields that are filled in with the activities pertaining to the individual (Figure 25). The information is collected through interviews with parents, professionals and others, depending on who is responsible for the activities at different times.

When filling in a day clock, it is necessary to ask about a

Figure 25. *Day clock for a twelve-year-old autistic boy.*

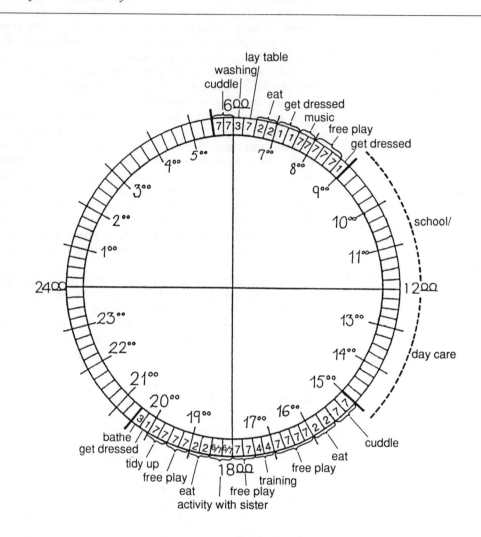

Situation	Code	Number	Time
Dressing/training	1	4	1
Eating	2	6	1.5
Washing/bathing	3	2	0.5
Training	4	2	0.5
Occupied alone	5	0	0
Occupied with children	6	2	0.5
Occupied with adults	7	20 (2)	5

typical day. It is a good idea to begin by asking about the previous day. If this was not a typical day, then one should ask about the last day that was suitably typical. The day clock can be divided into 15-minute intervals. Information is required about what the individual was doing and who was with him or her at every 15-minute interval. It is also useful when asking about each separate time period to ask whether any problems occurred in the situation, whether communication occurred, and if so, the type and manner of communication. It is a good idea to make two day clocks – one for normal weekdays, and one for normal weekends. When planning communication teaching, it may be an advantage to produce separate day clocks for communication. These will contain the times of the teaching situations, situations where the individual regularly communicates, and those where he or she sometimes communicates. In this way, it will become apparent when the person is not communicating.

A good day clock will give a picture of existing interventionary measures, the individual's activity level, activities that occur regularly and any problematical behaviour. This will include an overview of the total intervention, including daytime measures (nursery school, school, work or work-training), leisure activities and various forms of relief for caregivers. In addition, comprehensive interviews will give information about self-help skills, self-occupancy and communicative skills. When this information is pieced together with the routine tasks carried out by the family and other people in contact with the individual, one may get a picture of how the existing total intervention seems to work.

The day clock is used to find times that are suitable for communication teaching and other measures. As new activities are introduced, they are included in the day clock so that this will always show how the individual's day is organised. Thus, the day clock plays an important role in the ongoing evaluation of the intervention.

General skills

Interest in objects, activities and events

A basic principle that applies to the teaching of augmentative communication is that everyone wishes to communicate, but not everyone can. It has often been said that motivation on the part of the individual is a prerequisite for the implementation of teaching, but this raises the question of what it means not to be motivated. A lack of 'motivation' generally signals that the person appears negative and unwilling. There is no reason to take this as an expression of a general reluctance to communicate, but rather as an expression of the fact that the inability to do so is frustrating. Experience also shows that people become less reluctant and negative when they have learned some communication.

Even though everyone has a fundamental desire to communicate, they do not necessarily have a desire to communicate about anything and everything. If the teaching is to be successful, it is imperative that what is being taught is communication about things, activities and events about which the person is aware and interested in communicating. Assessment with regard to language teaching should therefore begin with an evaluation of the individual's interests.

In some cases it can be difficult to find things or activities that are interesting for the individual. When this is the case then measures must be taken to improve the situation: in such instances teaching should begin by creating interest and awareness.

Attention and initiation of communicative contact with others

Among people in need of augmentative communication, attention and initiation of communicative contact with others varies. This applies both within and between the main groups. The initiation of contact can be so unusual that only people who know the individual well can understand it. This can lead to the individual being strongly selective in terms of the people with whom he or she decides to initiate contact.

Within a 'pure' expressive language group, the ability to initiate contact with others may be deficient and perhaps non-existent. Some people do not have the physical qualifications to do anything that may be construed as a communicative initiative. The problem may also be due to the fact that they have only learned to answer others, not to take the initiative themselves; a form of learned dependence.

There is great variation among individuals in the supportive language group, but in this group also many individuals will show little motivation to initiate contact with others. The problems may be due to both learned dependency and the systematic unlearning of initiating contact on account of bad experiences. Many children in this group are shy and timid when they meet strangers, or may appear bothersome and aggressive. They may develop an aversion to speaking; or, in extreme cases, selective mutism, where they only speak to their close family (Helgevold, 1989).

It is in the alternative language group, however, that the most severe problems are found, both in terms of attention and initiation of communicative contact with others. This is probably related to the fact that these individuals generally have the poorest linguistic, communicative and social skills. The most distinctive sub-group in this respect is that of autistic children and adults, where problems in relating to other people are a diagnostic criterion. Initiation of contact and attention to others varies considerably within the group, however, and is dependent on the situation.

Self-help skills

Self-help skills include the ability to care for oneself, dress, wash, cook, etc. With the exception of very small children and people with very extensive motor disabilities, most people in need of augmentative communication possess some self-help skills. These skills comprise a significant part of the individual's opportunity of self-determination, and are of fundamental importance if the individual is to have any independence and private life. Self-help skills are generally discussed in interviews with people who know the individual, but it may also be useful to make observations of one's own. All three main groups have in common the fact that people around them often believe that they can do less than they are actually capable of doing.

In language and communication teaching it is important to take into account the need for self-help skills and, if possible, increase and facilitate training in these. As far as possible, language and communication teaching should be adapted to self-help training so that both forms of training are improved.

Self-occupancy

The extent to which the individual is able to occupy him- or herself determines how the intervention is arranged. Many families and other people in close contact with the individual find an inability to occupy him- or herself poses a considerable strain. Language and communication teaching may increase the degree of self-occupancy. In so far as an improved ability for self-expression may provide the individual with a better chance of choosing what he or she wants to do, good language and communication training may also improve the individual's initiative skills and reduce learned dependency on others.

Motor skills

The individual's motor skills are crucial for the choice of communication system and possible aids. The assessment of motor skills is twofold. First, the hand movements are assessed to determine whether or not the individual is able to use manual signs. In the case of those individuals who will have to use aided communication, the assessment is aimed at finding sitting positions and methods for pointing or activating switches.

It is clear that people with obvious motor disabilities are unable to use manual signs, but others may also have difficulty in performing these signs. However, it is important to distinguish between difficulty in producing manual signs due to motor disorders, and problems in following instructions. For example, it may be difficult for a mentally handicapped child to understand the idea of imitating a hand form. In the case of children with no obvious physical motor handicaps, it can be practical to take the performance of everyday skills as a starting point. The way these activities are carried out will also give cues as to how, if necessary, the signs can be simplified so that the individual is able to perform them (Figure 26).

If it has been decided that the individual will have to use a communication aid, it is imperative that the best possible method of pointing or activating a switch is found. This is often a difficult and time-consuming task, but it is essential if individuals with extensive motor disabilities are to be able to express themselves in the best possible way. There are some computer programs designed to assess motor functions, and there are also games and other programs designed to train individuals in the use of switches.

People with extensive motor disorders rely on a stable sitting position in order to use their motor skills. It is therefore important to find the sitting position that best facilitates pointing or activation of a switch.

Vision and hearing

Visual and auditory disorders are more common among all the three main groups than in the population in general. It is therefore important to have information about the individual's vision and hearing when a communication system is chosen and the training is planned. It is also vital that any problems the individual has with visual and auditory perception are made known to the assessor so that behaviour and test results can be appropriately interpreted. However, there are often difficulties testing the sight and hearing of many of the individuals in need of augmentative communication.

There are 'objective' tests for both sight and hearing, i.e. examinations that do not require cooperation on the part of the individual being examined. It is possible to examine whether the eye and ear are intact and in working order, and to register whether stimulation of the visual and auditory organs reach the brain. The last type of examination is not a reliable test for children with brain damage (cf. Rosenblum et al., 1980).

A seemingly intact sensory organ is no guarantee that the senses will function normally. Many mentally handicapped and autistic people appear to have sensory disturbances caused by brain damage. As a rule, these will not lead to deafness or blindness in the normal sense, since the person reacts to changes in stimulation, but the sense impressions will not be processed and perceived in a normal way. Objective examinations must therefore be supplemented by observations of how the individual actually uses vision and hearing.

Diagnosis

There are several good reasons for emphasising the necessity of an accurate diagnosis, even when this has no direct bearing on the planning of the intervention. In some cases the diagnosis is essential in order to provide the necessary medical treatment, but intervention is rarely a *direct* result of the diagnosis. Very often the measures that are implemented are general in the sense that they are provided for children and adults who belong to highly different diagnostic groups.

The most important reason for procuring a diagnosis is that this is often a means of securing the necessary intervention. The diagnostic label makes it easier to get support for the urgency of the intervention. For parents and others in close contact with the individual, the diagnosis can be necessary for obtaining realistic and tangible information about an individual's disorder. Information of this kind has often been given by parents of children with similar disorders, through organisations and through courses. The parents of disabled children arrange their own courses and also participate in courses that are open to both professionals and parents. The diagnosis provides contact with all these various sources of information.

A correct and accurate diagnosis is also necessary in order to make a prognosis, i.e. what may be expected based on previous experience. This applies both to professionals and to the individual's family.

There are many examples of a correct diagnosis of children and adults with language disorders helping to produce more suitable forms of intervention and improving the planning of such measures for future needs. For example, a girl may prove to have Rett's syndrome rather than being autistic as was previously assumed. This will mean that the intervention differs in a number of areas. The diagnosis may well lead to a move away from manual sign teaching, based on the assumption that the girl's motor skills will

Figure 26. *Everyday activities that can be used to assess motor skills (from Dennis et al., 1982).*

Hand form	pull trousers up/down	pull shirt up/down	squeeze oranges for juice	palm on table, pick up pencil in fingers	put on sock	squeeze toothpaste onto toothbrush	hold brush handle when brushing hair	crumple paper	wipe table with cloth or sponge	turn key	pick up book from table edge
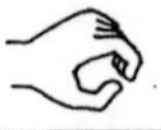 1 squeeze	x	x	x	x							
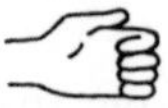 2 palmar						x	x	x			
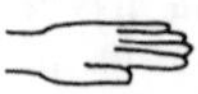 3 thumb adduction									x	x	x
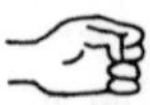 4 midposition of the forearm											
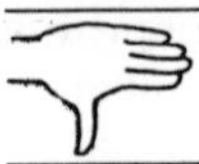 5 thumb abduction											
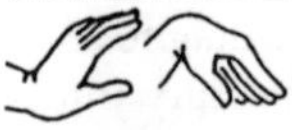 6 wrist movements							x				
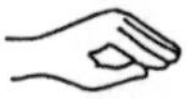 7 opposed grasp							x				
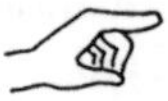 8 pointing radial finger											
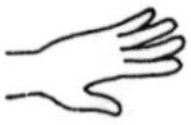 9 release											
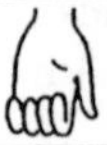 10 full supination											
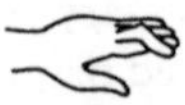 11 crossed finger											
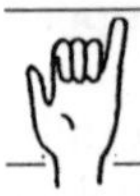 12 pointing ulnar finger											
Movement											
1 unilateral			x		x						
2 bilateral mirror	x				x						
3 unilateral across midline									x		
4 bilateral/one base—one mover						x					
5 bilateral two movers											
6 bilateral crossing midline											

self-feed using fingers/drink with cup	self-feed using utensils	turn steering wheel	hold sandwich or finger foods	hold jar of jam and twist lid	turn knobs/dials	comb hair	brush teeth	stir (contents in stable bowl)	pouring from container into glass held by other hand	button/unbutton	open and close zip on jacket	dial phone number	play instrument with keyboard	use finger puppet	wring wash cloth	tear paper	remove glove from fingers	retrieve object from pocket	throw ball up in air and catch
	x	x																	
			x	x	x	x	x												
						x	x	x											
										x	x	x	x	x					
											x	x							
																	x	x	
																			x
																	x		
x	x																		
x	x							x											
									x										
		x								x					x	x			

develop, to a communication board that the girl can use as long as she can point with her hands or eyes.

The family's need for support, relief and help

The families of individuals who need augmentative communication generally experience a great deal of strain. The degree of strain, and which pressures are greatest, depend on which group the child belongs to. The parents of children with severe motor disorders are normally subjected to a great deal of physical tension. Normal care and nursing is often time-consuming, and requires the individual to be lifted and moved frequently. For parents of autistic children, the pressures of always having to be present in order to prevent the child from injury, running away or damaging things, are often very great. What most families of children in need of augmentative communication have in common are the fact that everyday tasks become considerably more time-consuming than for others, that contact with other family members and friends is reduced, and that they are concerned about the future.

These strains imply that the family has a need for, and a right to, a reasonable amount of relief. How great this need is and how the relief should be organised will vary. The help must also be viewed in relation to the family's other tasks. In many instances day care for disabled children lasts only a short while during the middle of the day and there may be a need for some sort of help to cover the period from when the day care finishes to when the parents arrive home from work. The strain on the family may also be financial. Part of the total intervention is to ensure that the families are given the economic help and support they need and are entitled to, and that they are informed of their rights.

The ability to cope with these strains differs from family to family. In families where several individuals need much care and help (small children, sick or elderly family members), it is essential that resources be distributed. Some people are not as strong as others, and it is unreasonable to demand that everyone is as resourceful and robust as ideal parents might be. Experience shows that in many instances effective interventionary measures are not implemented because they place too great a strain on families that are given insufficient relief and help. A better relief system will make it easier to implement other measures.

The relief should not only depend on the immediate needs. Many families have a desire to fend for themselves and claim that they have little need for help, but over time the strain may nonetheless be too great. By ensuring that the family always has a reasonable amount of relief, it will also be more able to cope with pressures that arise later on.

Language and communication

Use

Most individuals who are about to start learning augmentative communication have little or no speech. The exception to this is children and adults who, because of motor disorders, have such unintelligible speech that it is useless in communication with anyone except those who know them well. An assessment of the individual's use of communication before language and communication teaching has begun will therefore usually be concentrated on forms of communication other than speech.

The form of communication used by children and adults in need of augmentative communication varies considerably. For children with severe motor disorders, the use of communication will, in some cases, be limited to looking at things in which they are interested, more or less articulated vocalisation as an expression of wishes and interests, crying, and other signs of excitement. Sometimes the strongest expression of interest is a change in muscle tonus, i.e. the child's body stiffens and stops making small movements.

Other children and adults with motor disorders and good language comprehension can often say 'yes' and 'no' by looking up and down, blinking, nodding and shaking their heads or by moving their heads in other ways. If children and adults with developmental disorders communicate in such a way, even while an assessment is being made of which first communication aid would be most appropriate, this means that they will receive the communication aid at too late a stage since they have already developed a considerable amount of language comprehension.

Children who belong to the alternative language group may also have very different forms of communication. However, a number of ways of communicating are common to many. The most usual form is that the child approaches an adult, takes hold of his or her hand and leads him or her to a place where there is something the child wants, or where a particular activity is usually carried out. This may, for example, be the refrigerator where a bottle of orange juice is usually kept. In instances of this kind the communication is typically composed of a succession of events. After the child and the adult have arrived at the refrigerator, the adult will open the refrigerator door and the child will reach out for the bottle of orange juice, perhaps at the same time saying 'uh, uh', or making other sounds.

Children who belong to the alternative language group may also use locations as part of their communication. There are children who sit down under the table when they want to go to the toilet, stand by the door to the kitchen when they are hungry, or sit down by their boots when they want to go out. These activities are also communicative expressions, but they may be difficult for adults and professionals to understand in the midst of their other daily tasks.

> Kathryn is an autistic 9-year-old girl. She is unable to speak. When her father drives the car into the garage, she often goes to the door and pulls at the door handle while she looks at her mother and makes a sound. In this way Kathryn expresses the fact that she wants to go for a drive with her father.

Children who have normal motor functions but who have not developed speech, use gestures in very different ways. Most children with specific language disorders will begin to use pointing as a form of communication. Autistic children, on the other hand, usually only use pointing when they have been specially taught to do so. However, the children in the supportive language group and the alternative language group often use idiosyncratic gestures that resemble words.

> Geoffrey is an 11-year-old autistic boy. He beats the table with his fist to say 'Daddy' (K. Steindal, personal communication 1990).

Idiosyncratic communication of this type is not only found among people with language and communication disorders. Similar communications are characteristic of the initial stages of speech development among children who develop language normally, and are usually called *vocables* (Ferguson, 1978). A vocable is defined as an articulation that has a fixed, recognisable acoustic form and a clearly defined use. Vocables have, however, no acoustic similarities with the conventional words. *Vroomvroom* can, for example, be used about toy cars and tractors, and *uvuvuv* about birds, aeroplanes, flies and other flying objects. Vocables and the equivalent gestures or utterances that are used by children with language disorders, have a use that does not correspond directly to specific words in the language. The fact that children do not use the words in the same way as adults is, however, a general feature of their language, and is not only linked to the use of vocables. A 1-year-old child may use *bow-wow* when speaking of dogs, cars and other machines, or say *dog* only when someone points at a picture of a dog.

The information given by the parents and others who are in daily contact with the child is the most important source of information about the various types of communication. This is a direct result of the fact that the communication often has a low frequency. The low incidence of communication means that usually only those people who are in close contact with the child have practical opportunities of knowing the form and extent of the communication.

A special problem for children with language disorders is that their idiosyncratic communication, which is the communication form they have that most resembles words, is often not recognised as 'proper' communication by teachers and other professionals. Parents also relate that they have not been believed when they have told others about this idiosyncratic communication.

Comprehension

It can be difficult to get a clear picture of what a person with pervasive language problems is able to understand. There are many examples where children and adults have been credited with a considerable understanding of speech, but careful observation has revealed that it was not the words they understood, but rather the gestures accompanying the speech, or special conditions in the situation.

> Martin is a 3-year-old autistic boy. He is very fond of going for walks, but does not react to the message 'Come on, let's go for a walk!' unless the nursery school teacher is simultaneously holding up his jacket or wearing her own coat (K. Steindal, personal communication 1990).

In some cases people with very extensive motor disorders may almost totally lack ordinary means of showing that they understand. Some people have for years been underestimated in terms of what they have understood both of speech, and of what has been going on around them. The underestimation has meant that these individuals have not been given the stimulation and the opportunities of development that they ought to have had.

> Joe Deacon lived in an institution for mentally handicapped people. He was considered to have no language until the age of 24. At that time another mentally handicapped inhabitant arrived who managed to interpret the sounds Joe made. Joe's abilities had to be totally re-assessed. Later, the two friends allied themselves with two other inhabitants, a mentally handicapped man who was able to use a typewriter and a physically handicapped wheelchair user who could spell. With the help of his friends, Joe wrote his autobiography, *Tongue Tied* (Deacon, 1974).

Less dramatic forms of underestimation frequently occur (cf. Fuller, Newcombe and Ounsted, 1983). It is difficult to use normal systematic observation with this group. Events that are most interesting will tend to occur rather infrequently. It would be impractical to carry out observations over such a long period. However, systematic observation can be used advantageously at the same time as training is started if it is carried out by those who are usually with the individual. The observations will then provide extra information about the individual's skills and will form the basis for evaluation and training.

The individual's capacity to express him or herself will, to a certain extent, also determine the methods that can be used to assess comprehension. If the individual can speak or write, and appears to have a reasonable vocabulary for self-expression, a good impression of language comprehension may be gained by asking various questions. It is much more difficult to assess comprehension when the individual has fewer words with which to demonstrate it. A person who can look up for *Yes* and down for *No* will be able to answer questions from ITPA such as: *Can tomatoes telegraph?* or: *Can mute musicians sing?* On the other hand, the person would not be able to complete another sub-test from ITPA, in which the task is to fill in sentences such as: *Mountains are high, valleys are ....*

For people who belong to the expressive language group, and others whom one knows to have a good understanding of language, tests can be useful tools if the person has the motor functions that are necessary to carry them out. A number of tests or test items place considerable demands on motor skills. For example, in Reynell's language scales (Reynell, 1969) the child has to carry out instructions such as: *Put the doll on the chair!* and: *Put all the pigs behind the brown horse!* Other tests are mainly based on pointing, but for many people with motor disabilities even pointing can be difficult to do precisely enough that another person can safely say which of several alternatives the person was pointing to. Some tests are specially adapted to children with motor disabilities; among others there is a language comprehension test for BBC computers (von Tetzchner, 1987).

However, the best information comes in the form of tangible reports from people who are in close contact with the person. These informants have the advantage of a wealth of experiences gained from being together with the person concerned. It is also these people, and the child's parents in particular, who, by spending so much time with the child or adolescent, have laid the foundations for the child's usage and understanding of language. The way the child demonstrates understanding can be very unusual and difficult for anyone other than the parents to discover. Nor are the parents always aware of the cues that they use. They are used to not being believed when they say that the individual is able to understand, but once the parents have been convinced that no one is interested in proving them wrong, systematic interviews can provide important information about the basis of the individual's comprehension. This information forms a base on which to build when it is time to begin planning intervention.

It is important to take one's time when speaking with those people who are in close contact with the individual. As a starting point, one may ask such questions as: *Think of something you are quite certain that you can say to John or make him understand in another way. What is it John does that makes you sure that he has understood you?* Questions of this kind can be asked in many different ways, and one should choose ones's words according to the needs of the person who is asked.

Parents or other people in contact with the child will usually begin by answering too generally. They may say things like: *I can tell just by looking at him.* It is important that the answers given are as specific as possible. General characterisations of the individual's language comprehension may well be correct, but may nonetheless be an insufficient basis for intervention. Follow-up questions are necessary. These may take the form of: *Yes, of course. But please describe it for me. What does he do? What does he look like when he's doing it? What is it he always understands? What is it he only seems to understand now and again?*

If the interviewer is patient, people in close contact with disabled people will almost always be able to answer questions of this type. It is our experience that this is also true of those in close contact with the lowest-functioning individuals.

A certain degree of over-interpretation is positive. However, the aim is to obtain the most correct picture possible of the individual's language comprehension. Overestimation means that the language teaching will not be adapted as well as it could be. It is especially easy to overestimate the language comprehension of a person who understands something of what is being said. For example, in a training or test situation one might say: *Point at the red ball*, whereby the person points correctly. It may be easy to immediately assume that the individual understands *everything* that is said. In addition, it is easy to imagine that the person can comprehend words that he or she understands in a given situation also in other, unrelated situations. This is often not the case. More extensive observation may reveal that the children understand only one or a few critical words in the sentence, and that they have learned to point in that particular situation.

Martin is a 3-year-old autistic boy. He is fond of orange juice, and usually comes running when his mother shouts: 'Come and have some orange juice'. His mother was told to shout out in the same way as usual but sit still without moving. She was quite surprised to find that Martin did not react, but carried on twirling a toy. A short while later she stood up, walked toward the kitchen table where the bottle of orange juice was standing and repeated the words. Martin came running immediately (K. Steindal, personal communication 1990).

Understanding what is going on in communicative situations depends not only on what is being said with the aid of signs or speech. There are many conditions that contribute to our understanding of a situation and give cues as to what is probably being said. The rattling of pots and pans in the kitchen may indicate that someone is cooking, holding a coat may indicate that someone is soon to leave the house, etc. In addition, what is being said is often accompanied by eye contact, pointing and other gestures, and this contributes to the understanding of the situation, even if what is being said is not in itself understood.

Likewise, one may observe that individuals only show they understand when in the company of certain people. One should nonetheless be wary of concluding that the individuals do not understand anything of what is being said. Among many people in need of augmentative communication, their understanding of single words or expressions may depend on the situation.

The fact that an individual's understanding of speech is linked to the use of gestures or other types of non-verbal communication will, in many cases, not be apparent in interviews with those in close contact with the individual. The person who participates in the communicative situation will not normally be aware of this. Systematic observation of the communicative situation is therefore necessary when the information provided gives the impression that the communication is dependent on a situation or person. Documentation of such dependency can be a good starting point for further discussion about the teaching with parents and others in contact with the child.

Information about how the parents and others judge the individual's comprehension also has another function. It provides cues as to how people interpret the individual's comprehension, how they react to his or her means of expressing this comprehension, and the extent to which they try to adapt their own communication so that comprehension can be improved. This knowledge will be useful when assessing the language environment and adapting it so that it encourages the best possible acquisition of linguistic and communicative skills.

Evaluating the language intervention

There should be continual evaluation of the intervention on the basis of the objectives. Regardless of how well one plans in advance, one cannot take for granted that the development will be as assumed. It is therefore important that the evaluation is planned beforehand and is included as a part of the intervention right from the beginning of the teaching. Planned evaluation will help clarify the teaching objectives and make it easier to see the relationship between the different teaching aims. Since the evaluation is planned, the intervention does not have to be clearly inappropriate before it is adjusted or modified.

An evaluation should be as extensive as is practically possible. It should cover the specific aims that have been set for the language teaching, and also evaluate the generalised effects of the teaching in terms of the total life situation, i.e. whether the person shows fewer behavioural problems, is more social, participates in more activities, is more attentive during the training, etc.

Specific goals

The evaluation of the language teaching should include information about the progress in terms of the specific teaching goals and the signs that have been taught. This means a registration of the use of signs and the development of other linguistic and communicative skills that are being taught. The specific goals can be the use of new signs, sentences or contact strategies, a higher level of linguistic activity, etc.

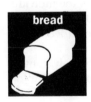

The individual does not necessary learn what has been stated as the teaching aim. Sometimes the teaching situation has been such that the individual has learned a use other than the one that was planned. This is not necessarily negative.

> Giles is a mentally handicapped boy of 19. He was trained to use the sign BREAD, but quickly began to use the sign as a general call for help and to express that there was something he wanted. This usage of the sign was extremely functional for him, and instead of forcing him to use it 'correctly', BREAD was redefined as 'HELP'.

This example emphasises how necessary it is to not merely register 'right' and 'wrong', but also to analyse the pattern of usage and understanding of the sign and find a possible fixed usage that was not intended by the teacher. If, in the example above, Giles's teacher had insisted that the sign retain the meaning she had tried to teach him, this would have taken away the communication he had acquired. By continually evaluating the situation, it is possible to adapt to

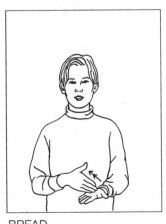

BREAD

an unexpected development when this is most functional.

In the evaluation the report should also include the type and extent of help that is needed at any given time for the individual to accomplish a specific communicative act in the teaching situation. The teaching may can be carried out in a number of ways, and reduction in the amount of help needed should always be a basic aim. In reports about sign teaching it is common to merely indicate the number of signs that are being practised or are in use. An evaluation may show considerable progress, despite the fact that the individual has not begun to learn and use new signs because the amount of help has been reduced.

Generalised effects

Other skills besides linguistic and communicative abilities should also be included in the evaluation because the different skills influence one another. New language skills bring with them new information about the surroundings, learning of concepts, and social skills in the broadest sense (cf. Konstantareas, Webster and Oxman, 1979). Likewise the understanding of and experience in mastering different activities will be related to the individuals' ability to understand the communication of others and be able to express themselves. Successful language and communication training has great consequences for a large number of activities. In general, it may be said that those aspects of the individual's general life situation that were included in the assessment before the training should also be included in the evaluation.

The evaluation of the training should not only contain reports about the training situation, but also include information about the use of language in the home and other situations. It is especially important that spontaneous use of signs is registered. However, there are different forms of spontaneous use. Spontaneous use may mean that the person uses signs that have not been practised in the teaching situation. These signs will perhaps be construed as wrong with regard to the training, but they may represent genuine attempts at communication. Spontaneous use may mean that the person uses the sign on request outside of the teaching situation or that the person takes the initiative and uses the sign without help. The reports should also contain information about the type of help that may be given for what is called spontaneous use.

The evaluation of the language teaching should also contain information about which objects, activities and events each sign is used to communicate: for example, whether the signs are used to communicate about objects or activities other than those that exist within the training

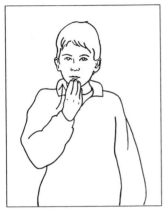

EAT

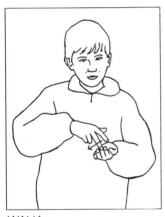

WALK

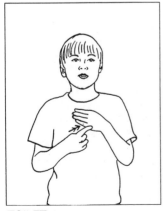

TOILET

situation. One needs to know whether the individual uses the sign in a wider sense than is normal (overextension), or whether the sign is used in a more restricted way, i.e. about a smaller set of activities and objects than is usual (underextension).

A coordination of language and communication training with other training goals implies that the language training can only to a small extent be seen in isolation. The evaluation must include those areas of life and functions that were the point of departure for choosing the specific training goals. For children and adults with motor disorders, this may entail an assessment of the extent to which the training has led to more conversations, and the extent to which the person has gained more control over the content of the conversations.

Information transfer when changing school, work and home

A large number of people who receive augmentative communication have a need for intervention that is not limited by time. For those people in the expressive language group who have extensive motor disorders, new environments must be organised as they pass through new phases of life. Communication aids are being developed that create new possibilities, but they require that the individuals and those around them undergo training in how to use these aids. In the alternative language group the acquisition of new skills is often slow, and the need for training will continue throughout life. This means that the training will take place in different environments as the individual changes school, work and home. Children in the supportive language group, who are given training in augmentative communication for only a limited period of time, may also change their school or home environment.

When a person with an organised environment and training moves, it is crucial that there are routines for the transferral of information from those in charge of the training and organisation to those who are to assume responsibility. All too often these routines are lacking, which results in discontinuity in the training and loss or stagnation in the development of skills.

Raymond is a mentally handicapped 20-year-old boy. He receives special education at a high school. He follows simple instructions, but he neither speaks nor uses signs. According to his notes, he received training in manual signs from the age of 13. By the time he was transferred to another school at the age of 16, he had learned to use the signs EAT, WALK and TOILET, and was learning several new signs. When he was 18 he was transferred to a new

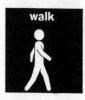

school, and in the notes that were transferred with him it said that 'he was in the process of learning to use signs'. At the age of 19 he changed school again. When he changed school at the age of 20, the teacher sent with him a list of over 50 signs that Raymond had been given teaching in and comments as to how they were executed. It was not apparent, however, whether Raymond had used any of the signs spontaneously. Thus, after six years of teaching Raymond uses no signs spontaneously (Kollinzas, 1984).

There is every reason to believe that Raymond's lack of skills is related to his changing schools and the discontinuity he experienced in training. Kollinzas (1984) has devised a *communication record* for the registration of communication skills and training, which can be used for the transferral of this type of information (Figure 27). The record contains the information that *must* be included when the person changes training environment; i.e. the gloss of the signs that are used, a description of how the person performs or points out the signs, and a description of the situations in which each sign occurs.

The communication record will help give the people in the new environment realistic expectations of the individual and to organise the situation as well as possible. It will also help to uncover the need for training of people in the environment to which the person moves. Usually, it is useful to have some guidance from the professionals who have worked with the individual before the move. In many instances of augmentative communication intervention, external consultants and instructors are also used. The communication record will make it possible for the professionals who take over to assess whether it is desirable and possible to use the same external consultants for guidance and training in the new environment.

Some of the individuals with communication disorders who have acquired some linguistic skills may themselves be able to help in the training of new environments and new people who arrive in their environment.

Isabel is a 13-year-old girl with Down's syndrome. She uses approximately 70 manual signs spontaneously, and does not have intelligible speech. Her teacher has made a folder with drawings of all the manual signs she uses. The gloss of the sign is written above the drawing. New signs are included as Isabel learns them. Isabel carries this book with her wherever she goes. When new personnel or helpers appear Isabel sits with them and works through the book. Isabel shows how the signs are performed while the new helper struggles to learn them. This is a change of roles that Isabel clearly appreciates (K. Steindal, personal communication 1990).

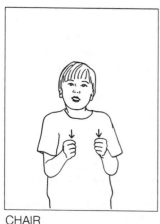

CHAIR

It is both unfair toward the person and a poor use of resources if what has been learned is not maintained and

igure 27. *Communication record*
from Kollinzas, 1984).

COMMUNICATION RECORD

Name : Per Hansen	*Sign system*	*Code*
Age: 13;7	Pictogram	P
Instructor: Hans Larsen	Manual signs	H
Place: Vik school		
Date: 2–10–88		
Page: 2 of 4		

Sign	System	Execution	Situation information
CHAIR	H	Normal	Performs the sign when the teacher shows the picture
TABLE	H	Normal	Performs the sign when the teacher shows the picture
KICK	P		Points himself in order to select the activity in the gymnasium
HORSE	H	Right hand between middle and ring finger	Executed alone when he knows he is going to ride
TOILET	H	Normal	Uses the sign spontaneously sometimes when he wants to go to the toilet. He is hand-guided to perform the sign when he is taken to the toilet
DOOR	H	Normal	Uses the sign spontaneously when he wants to go out
TELEVISION	P		Uses spontaneously at home when he wants to watch television
BOOTS	H	Indistinct	Not used spontaneously, the sign is hand-guided during dressing
SCARF	H	Indistinct	Not used spontaneously, the sign is hand-guided during dressing

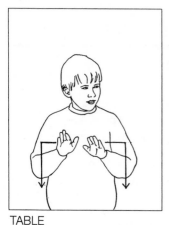

TABLE

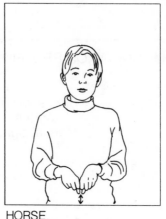

HORSE

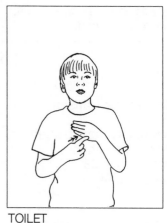

TOILET

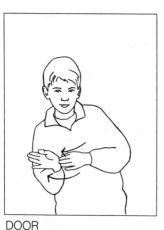

DOOR

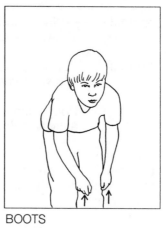

BOOTS

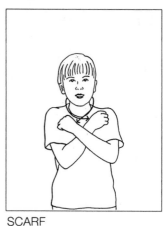

SCARF

built upon. The transferral of information that can min-
imise the negative effects of a change in the training and living environment is therefore of great significance. For those
who have been in charge of training the person, the filling
in of the communication record will be a part of the planning of the transferral. For those who assume responsibility,
it will be a part of the assessment of the individual.

Defining areas of responsibility

In working for disabled individuals, experience has shown
that the quality of the individual measures is to a large
degree dependent on the presence of and quality of other
interventionary measures. Experience has also shown that it
can be difficult to ensure coherence and continuity in the
interventionary measures. The measures that most generally cause problems are those administered by several help
authorities, and to start with it is often unclear who has

responsibility for the various areas. Experience shows that when things go wrong and the person does not get the necessary intervention, this is often the result of unclear areas of responsibility and a lack of coordination. This lack of coordination is even more clearly visible in long-term plans for intervention. The more extensive the disorder, the greater the need for both long-term and short-term planning in order to ensure that the measures that are given are in proportion to the present and future needs of the individual. It is therefore crucial that the individual measures are seen in terms of a total goal, and that a major plan is drawn up for the measures in which the areas of responsibility for the total intervention and the individual measures are clarified.

It has gradually been recognised that the need for coordination and planning is central in the care of disabled people. This means that the financial responsibility must be allocated, likewise the responsibility for coordinating the various elements of the intervention and ensuring that they are seen in terms of a sensible long-term plan. There should be one person who knows all the measures well, and who can act as a care manager, and whom the family and the other professionals involved can contact. It is also useful to have routines for the implementation of new initiatives. When things go wrong this is often due to the fact that no one feels responsible for taking the initiative to implement the required modifications.

In order to fill this need, *responsibility groups* have gradually been established. The groups are multi-disciplinary, and which professionals will participate depends on the intervention required. Together the group should have a complete overview of the intervention, be able to initiate new measures and distribute the various forms of responsibility.

Chapter 6
The teaching situation

Children and adults who are taught augmentative communication have been unable to acquire sufficient language and communicative skills in a normal environment. They are dependent on the fact that the environment is specially organised for them.

For the alternative language group and the supportive language group, the primary object of this organisation is to create appropriate teaching situations. The purpose of organising the environment is that the new form of communication must be learned and used. The expressive language group does not have the same need for language teaching. In cases where language comprehension is good, the main aim is to organise the environment so that it *facilitates* communication and the natural acquisition and use of language. In reality, this means providing a communication aid and the largest possible vocabulary that is accessible in all situations, and making it easier for others to understand what is being expressed.

People in the expressive language group experience many situations during the course of a normal day where it is impossible for them to communicate with others. The aim of facilitating communication is to remedy this and thereby enable the individual to experience increased participation in everyday activities. The need for teaching is mainly limited to the youngest children in the expressive language group and – for the older children – to an introductory phase in which the system and signs that are to be used are explained. Teaching reading and writing is such an introductory phase.

Designing the teaching situation

It is usual to distinguish between *special training* and training in *natural situations*. In special training the person who is being taught is taken out of the normal environment. Specific teaching procedures and goals have been formulated. The signs that are to be practised, the time and place for training, the people present and the material that is to be used; everything is planned in advance. When the teaching takes place in 'natural situations', it occurs in the environment in which the individual is usually found, and the teaching of specific signs is often linked to situations where it is believed or known that the individual will have a use for the sign.

There is no clear dividing line between special training and training in natural situations. The degree of organisation can vary considerably even though the teaching takes place in the individual's normal environment. It is therefore appropriate to distinguish between *planned* and *spontaneous* teaching in natural situations. In planned teaching a specific teaching goal has always been decided in advance. In addition to which signs or sign constructions that are to be taught, time, location, material to be used, and who is to give the training may vary – but at least one of these has been planned. If all this is planned the only difference between planned teaching in natural situations and special training is that the teaching occurs in a location where the individual can usually be found. In addition, a training situation so meticulously planned that it alters what the individual is used to can hardly be called a 'natural' situation.

Spontaneous teaching situations are characterised by a small degree of organisation. It is generally a matter of being aware of the individual's use of specific signs, and perhaps of providing opportunities in which these signs can be used. In some cases the teaching goal – for example, to teach the use of a specific sign – is decided beforehand, but the training can also take place without this having been planned, merely because an opportunity suddenly presents itself.

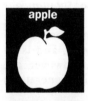

At fixed times Jack is taken to a room in his nursery school that is used for individual training. Here he practises APPLE, BANANA and ORANGE. Two teachers take turns at teaching him. This is special training.

Three times a day Jack is allowed to choose between apple and banana or between apple and orange. The teaching takes place in the part of the nursery school where they usually eat, immediately before the normal meal. He is allowed to choose 10 small pieces of fruit so that he is not too full up before his meal. This is meticulously planned teaching in a natural environment.

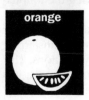

Every day at 2 p.m. the children eat fruit in the nursery school. Because Jack is learning to choose between apple, banana and orange, his teachers have made sure that the bowl of fruit contains only two types of fruit, which must be apple, banana or orange. This type of training may be regarded as one with a small

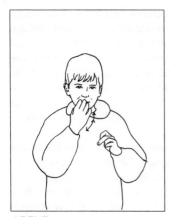

APPLE

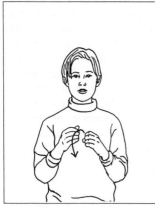

BANANA

degree of planning or as slightly planned spontaneous teaching.

The nursery school leaves a tray of fruit with apples, bananas and oranges on a table in the afternoon. If Jack tries to make a sign or approach someone in order to get fruit, the situation is used to allow him to use the signs. This is spontaneous learning.

There is no clash of interests between the teaching in natural situations and special training. The choice to carry out teaching in specially planned situations in which the individual is not otherwise found, depends on the teaching goal. An evaluation of the individual's preferences, needs and abilities determines this and the easiest way of achieving it. In general, special training and teaching in natural situations occur at the same time. Planned teaching in the natural environment should be just as well prepared as special training. This implies among other things that specific teaching goals are formulated and the motivation and attention of the individual who is to learn is secured. At the same time it is important to stress that skills learned are not automatically good or useful merely because the teaching has taken place in a normal environment. The signs that are practised should have an obvious utility value for the individual in question or for the surroundings.

Planning for generalisation

In the teaching of manual and graphic signs *generalisation* means that the individual uses the signs *spontaneously* to describe new objects, in combinations with new words or signs, in new situations, or with new people. *Spontaneous use* means that the individual uses the sign without being prompted to do so. Spontaneous use may also occur both in training situations and in new situations, and is an important goal in language intervention. However, the main aim is simultaneous spontaneous and generalised use.

It is important to distinguish between generalisation and *teaching extended use*. If the individual, having learned to use a sign in one specific situation, undergoes successful training in the use of the sign in relation to new objects, combinations, situations or people, this is called extended use. The extended use is not in itself an expression of generalisation, but it may be instrumental in laying the foundations for later generalisation.

Many people who belong to the alternative language or supportive language groups have problems in transferring learning from the training situation to other situations. This is termed the 'problem of generalisation'. For example, it is rare for an autistic child who has learned to use a sign in a

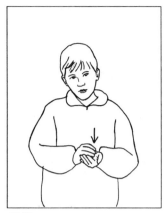

CUP

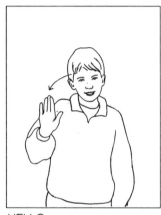

HELLO

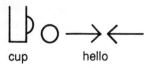

cup   hello

special training situation to begin to use it unprompted in new situations. In addition, there are many individuals – especially in the alternative language group – who need a long time to learn. Both of these circumstances call for locating the training in situations where the learned skills are to be used.

Traditionally, little attention has been paid to generalisation in language training. The main emphasis has been on learning the form itself; it was assumed that generalisation would more or less follow automatically once the execution of the sign had been learned.

When language instruction is given in special training situations, it is essential that plans have been made in advance as to how to solve the problem of transferring new skills to other situations. One of the most common methods is to include elements from those situations where the communication will be used, i.e. making the special training situation resemble the natural situation more closely. In order to do this effectively, it is important that before starting one has a detailed knowledge of the situations to which one intends to transfer the skills. During the planning of special training situations it often becomes clear that it is just as expedient to begin with planned teaching in the natural environment without preliminary special training. Thus, planning for the transferral of skills to natural situations ensures that special training is used only when there are strong arguments in favour of doing so.

Just as there are strategies for the transferral from special training situations to natural situations, there must also be strategies for making planned situations less organised. During the planning of these strategies, it may also become evident that the natural situations can be accomplished with less organisation than was first assumed.

Training in extended use has also been used as a way of facilitating generalisation. Less limitation of the training situations may lead to increased generalisation. In order to promote the generalisation to new objects, it has been suggested that several different exemplars of the same class of objects should be used. This means that when practising the sign CUP, one should use cups of different shapes, sizes and colours. Skills that are trained with only one teacher are often not transferred to other people. The generalisation to new people may be facilitated if several people carry out the same teaching. Sometimes it may be sufficient for two people to carry out the training, so that the individual understands that the skill can be used in several different situations. Stokes, Baer and Jackson (1974), for example, trained mentally handicapped children to say hello, but discovered that the children said hello only to the teacher that trained them. After two teachers began to take turns at teaching, the children began to say hello to the whole staff of 20 people.

Duration and location of the teaching sessions

When language and communication teaching is woven into and becomes an integral part of the normal activities, the duration of the teaching will dictate itself. With planned teaching in natural situations, the duration may vary, but the sessions should be short, preferably 5–10 minutes, and be repeated several times each day. It is more important that the teaching is functional than that it is repeated many times. Special teaching situations should also be spread throughout the day. It is often practical to have individual sessions that last longer, but not so long so that the individual becomes bored or tired. Gradually, the teaching times can be varied, so that no unnecessary dependence on time is created.

It is sometimes out of consideration for the professionals involved that the situations become more organised.

> Kerry is a 5-year-old autistic girl. She is always taught by a special teacher in natural situations. The teaching takes place at fixed times, depending on the special teacher's itinerary. As part of the reduction in planning, the nursery school teacher and assistant are given guidance in how they can carry out short training sessions. Thus, Kerry will receive more teaching and this will be more varied in terms of times and persons, which in turn will foster generalisation of the skills she learns.

Flexible teaching strategies, which, in so far as it is possible, utilise natural situations, place demands on the organisation of teaching. In particular, professionals who are not directly connected to the individual's nursery school, school or day-care centre, will find themselves having to work more indirectly, i.e. by supervising and teaching those who work in the individual's everyday environment.

Structuring

The terms structure and structuring are used in different ways and have no generally accepted definition. They are often used fairly loosely to indicate that the intervention designed for an individual undergoing training is planned and that, to a certain extent at least, the activities that occur during the day are planned. Structuring is a useful tool for obtaining an overview of and organising the day so that the activities play a part in promoting training in the use and understanding of language and communication. In order to be able to analyse the structure of a 24-hour period, it is necessary to distinguish between the various levels of structuring. In the following a distinction is made between *frame structure*, *situational structure* and *cues*.

Frame structure

Frame structure is the division into different *situations*, i.e. routines, events, activities, etc., that make up one day. Thus, a day always has a frame structure, whether it is planned or not. Producing an overview of a normal day for the learner means assessing the frame structure that exists before the teaching is implemented. An assessment of the frame structure provides a basis for obtaining a relatively simple overview of how the activities are spread out during the course of the day, how long the different activities last, and what proportion of the individual's waking day is planned. The assessment also gives information about how many of the different activities are repeated daily, and how fixed the daily itinerary is. This is basic information for the evaluation of the total intervention and the planning of language and communication teaching.

Weekdays may be more or less similar, and the frame structure filled up to different degrees. The frame structure also includes the total intervention. It is therefore the total life situation and the need for teaching and function that should govern what is included in the future frame structure. An ordinary weekday should consist of teaching sessions, social intercourse, everyday routines, leisure activities and periods of relaxation.

What distinguishes a planned frame structure from a casual one is generally the range of fixed activities that are included in situations that are repeated at fixed intervals. The frame structure can be made more dense by filling in the periods of time in which nothing much happens with new activities. A planned and dense frame structure can be a useful tool for language and communication teaching. This applies particularly to the alternative language group. For those who profit from a dense frame structure, the teaching should, in principle, be organised in 15-minute sessions although some situations may last longer than this. This means that for each 15-minute period throughout the day a note should be made of what is going to happen, and the aim of each individual activity should be formulated. In reality the frame structure will not always be followed completely: some flexibility is needed in order to take account of unforeseen events and the family's need for variation.

For the expressive language group, assessment of frame

structure usually has a function other than that of planning the teaching. The lives of the people who belong to this group consist mostly of routines with little variation and flexibility. Daily routines, such as morning toilet and breakfast, can take a long time, and often the day consists of little other than the fixed activities. There is a lot of free time, and the individual is only to a limited extent able to determine what will happen. Many people with motor disorders are not very mobile and depend on a vehicle for mobility and a helper to accompany them. An assessment of the frame structure of school-age children will usually reveal a great need for help outside school hours. Such help with leisure-time activities and social intercourse with peers is often given little priority, and the result is that the children are at home for most of their leisure time. This hampers their chances of participating in social activities and developing independence and positive self-esteem.

When assessing the frame structure in the day of a disabled child, it may be a useful exercise to make a similar assessment of the frame structure in the day of a child of similar age living in the same environment. A comparison of this kind will not only show the differences in their lives, but also provide ideas for activities that can be introduced for the disabled child.

Situational structure

The different situations that make up a frame structure also have their own built-in structure. This is what is called situational structure. Since the situations have varying degrees of organised content, it is possible to speak of varying degrees of structuring. In those situations with least structuring, matters such as where the person will be, who will be present, or which activities will be take place, are undecided. In the most highly structured situations, everything is decided in advance, and the situation also has a defined teaching goal.

A large degree of structuring will give an overview that enables one to be systematic. For those responsible for the teaching, a fixed and dense situational structure enables them to teach more effectively. The aim of the structuring is to make it easier to know what should be done in the situation; i.e. how one should react, create expectations for the individual in terms of what is going to happen, organise the communication and plan how to expand the language training.

Cues

Cues enable people to understand what another person is communicating. In principle, the number of possible cues is infinite, since communication may take place in so many individual ways and in different situations. In communication with people who are unable to speak, the cues that help comprehension may be activities that are carried out, objects in the surroundings, something that happens in the situation, cultural norms, what one usually does, etc.

> Angela is a 12-year-old girl with Rett's syndrome. When she heard her grandfather's voice from the room next door, she turned her gaze to a book. This was understood to be her way of communicating that she wanted her grandfather to read for her – a common occurrence. In this situation both the grandfather's voice and the fact that the girl looked at the book were cues that made such an interpretation reasonable.

In general, cues may be described in terms of individuals' tendency to react to behaviour as though it were communicative. It is the presence of cues to communication that makes people react to a given behaviour as though it were communication.

When cues have been described or planned in advance they form part of the situational structure. The description of the cues to comprehension in a situation can thus be regarded as a third level of structuring. An assessment of the use of communication in an individual who is to learn augmentative communication is largely an assessment of cues. In language and communication intervention it may often be fruitful to ask questions about how a teaching situation can be structured by building cues into a situation. This means that, in addition to teaching the individual, manual signs for instance, the situation is also arranged so that it contains elements that make the communication reasonable and understandable.

Initiating the intervention

For all children in need of augmentative communication, it is important that the teaching begins as early as possible. The most important argument for this is that there appears to be a sensitive period for language acquisition; i.e. it is easier for children of pre-school age to learn language than it is for older children and adults. This same also applies to augmentative communication.

The existence of a sensitive period seems probable for several reasons. Observations of small children show that they can quickly learn a foreign language without a trace of an accent, while older children and adults have difficulties in shedding their own accent. Brain damage that leads to language disorders in adults produces fewer or none of the same effects in children. Newborn babies who have had their left brain hemisphere removed – as is the case with Siamese twins joined together at the head – have learned to speak normally (Lenneberg, 1967). Children with a severe hearing impairment who are fitted with a hearing aid so that they can perceive language sounds show fewer deviations from normal speech if they begin using a hearing aid at a very early age (Fry, 1966).

On the basis of investigations of people with poorly developed language, there appears to be an important dividing line around the age of 4–5 years in terms of speech acquisition. The proportion of people with mental handicap who learn to speak does not appear to increase after this age. It is generally claimed that the chances of a child developing speech are very poor if he or she has not begun to speak before the age of 5 years (Rutter, 1985). It should be stressed, however, that there are people who have begun to speak later than this, and who have developed some speech without the use of augmentative communication. There are also examples of adolescents and adults without speech who have begun to speak later, after being taught augmentative communication.

The effect of sign teaching on speech acquisition

The teaching of signs is often begun at too late a stage. This is due to a number of reasons, but fear that teaching a child to use manual or graphic signs will hinder the development of speech has been one significant reason. This fear has led people to defer the augmentative communication until traditional speech training has proved to be a failure (Carr, 1988; Wells, 1981).

The discussion about the relationship between signs and speech has its origins in the teaching of deaf people, where this discussion over the last two centuries has had very emotional overtones (cf. Lane, 1984). One stubborn myth is that sign teaching can hinder the development of speech. There is no research showing that the acquisition of sign language has a negative effect on the development of speech. On the contrary, a number of investigations show that signs have positive effects on speech. For example, the non-deaf children of deaf parents develop both sign language and speech, and are thus fully bilingual (Prinz and Prinz, 1979, 1981).

Many of those who were given language instruction were people who had undergone several years of speech training without appreciable results. Some of these individuals have begun to speak after first learning to use manual or graphic signs (Casey, 1978; Romski et al., 1988). This reinforces the assumption that different communication skills influence and enhance one another.

Because speech and augmentative communication may support one another, augmentative communication should be taught as early as possible. In the case of children who are at risk of not developing speech normally, it is natural to implement intervention before the problems become apparent, thereby preventing the negative effects of poor communication and encouraging the development of communicative skills.

Chapter 7
Teaching strategies

The need for the adaptation of teaching methods to suit individuals is universally recognised. However, it is common practice for many children and adults with different types of disorders to receive the same teaching. In our opinion the lack of a distinction between the teaching goals and methods for individuals with different impairments poses a major problem in the field of augmentative communication. The object of this work is therefore not to give ready-made 'recipes'. Instead we wish to review the *principles* and methods of teaching. Some of these principles and methods are based on theory, others are based on our own and others' experiences. The teaching aims and methods used should vary from individual to individual, and selection of these should be based on practical considerations. A variety of methods be used, and these should be governed by principles and experience, adapted to the practical circumstances and in line with the total intervention.

There are a variety of ways of teaching sign use. Most of these methods have been recognised and used for a long time. From time to time, however, new variations of recognised teaching strategies are presented that give rise to trends and ideological debate. In this chapter a number of different strategies are presented, some of them very similar, some of them less so. The purpose of classifying the strategies is to bring out the fact that different strategies presuppose varying degrees of planning, structure and knowledge about the learner. The strategies are not mutually exclusive, and can often be used in parallel. They have different strengths and weaknesses, and some will thus suit one disabled individual better than another.

Comprehension and use of signs

In the following a distinction is made between teaching directed at an individual's *use* of signs and *comprehension*

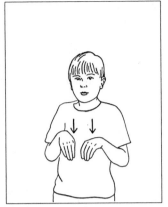

FATHER

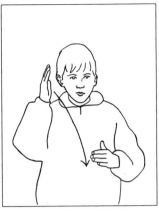

WAIT

STOP

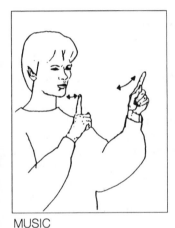

MUSIC

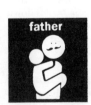

father

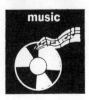

music

of signs. In *comprehension training* the conversational partner addresses him- or herself to the learner. The individual has to learn to understand the manual or graphic signs and either answer what has been said or perform an activity to demonstrate understanding. It is the conversational partner who points at or performs the signs.

In the early stages of learning most of the signs used in comprehension training are *signal signs* or *command signs. Signal signs* are those signs that indicate subsequent activities and events, and are used by the conversational partner to give information to the learner. Signal signs may be performed by the teacher using either the individual's hands or the teacher's own hands to perform the manual sign or point at the graphic sign.

> Philip is a mentally handicapped 23-year-old. He lives in a community unit, where his father usually visits him every Saturday. Before his father enters his room, one of the staff members makes the sign FATHER while simultaneously saying the word father.

Command signs are signs used by the conversational partner to get the learner either to carry out an activity or to stop one. These signs are pointed at or performed by the conversational partner. WAIT may be a particularly useful command sign.

> David is an autistic boy of 7. He can stand for long periods of time switching the light on and off. His teacher uses the sign STOP while saying stop emphatically in order to make him refrain from what he is doing.

Expressive signs are manual and graphic signs that are made by the individual when he or she addresses another person as a means of achieving a particular goal, informing about a specific event, commenting on an activity, etc.

Training use implies the teaching of the signs' functional use. The object of the teaching is to get the individual to initiate communication with the conversational partner. The conversational partner must understand the signs and answer the individual or react to them appropriately. During the teaching the individual may be given help to perform manual signs or point at graphic signs, but only where necessary.

> Mary is a 14-year-old mentally handicapped girl. She likes to listen to music and is learning the sign MUSIC in a special teaching situation. There are two teachers. A cassette player is placed on the table out of her reach. When she tries to reach it, one of the teachers guides her hands to make the manual sign MUSIC. The other teacher gives her the cassette player and she is allowed to listen to one melody.

Teaching comprehension

Natural situations

Many individuals with the most severe language and communication disorders have no overview of what their day will contain in terms of activities and events. They are often taken passively from one activity to another without being told what is going to happen. Nor do they take the initiative in starting an activity, or showing whether or not they like what has been planned for them. Their reaction to this feeling of uncertainty about what is happening often results in anxiety or fear; they become passive or inactive, or resist when someone wants them to take part in something new.

> Martin is a 3-year-old autistic boy. Every time he has to change activity in his nursery school and go to another room he lies down on the floor, kicking his legs and crying. It takes a long time to quieten him down. His day at nursery school is marked by these problems (K. Steindal, personal communication 1990).

One of the primary objectives of communication training of individuals who are unable to decide for themselves what they are going to do is that they can at the very least be told *what* is going to happen. One way of achieving this is to design a tight frame structure in which activities occur in the same place, at the same time and in the same order, and where routine activities are signalled with the help of *markers*. This approach may be called *marker-controlled frame structuring*.

The marker that is chosen should be easy for the learner to recognise, and it should be presented immediately before the activity begins. It is also useful if a marker is used to indicate when the activity is finished. In principle

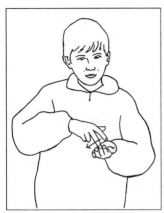

WALK

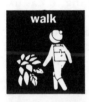

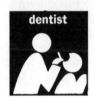

markers may be anything; for example, manual signs performed with the individual's hands, graphic signs, objects that are used in the activities, etc. Using manual or graphic signs is the best strategy because this will simultaneously lead to language learning. No matter whether signs, objects or other markers are used, marker-controlled frame structuring is a form of comprehension training. The aim is that the individual will learn that the markers precede specific activities and events, i.e. that they function as signals. Markers may signal both positive and negative events.

> John is a 10-year-old multi-handicapped boy who seems to like being taken out for walks in his wheelchair. Before he is taken out, he is guided to point at the PIC sign WALK.

> Marie is a 17-year-old mentally handicapped girl. She has very bad teeth and is often at the dentist. Before she visits the dentist, who is situated in the building next door, she is guided to make the sign DENTIST.

Like many other people, Marie is afraid of visiting her dentist. If she is informed where she is going before each visit to the dentist, she will not be afraid of walking in the direction of the dentist's surgery on occasions when she is not going to visit the dentist. As she gradually begins to understand what the sign signals, she will begin to protest when a member of staff makes the sign DENTIST, but she will nonetheless go along – albeit reluctantly.

The clearest indication that the marker has begun to have a signal function is that the individual begins to anticipate what is going to happen. Among individuals with the most severe forms of impairment, this may manifest itself in straightening up, becoming more excited, or showing increased muscle tonus when the marker is presented. Gradually the person may perhaps begin to look in the direction of, or move toward the place, where the activity takes place, or where specific things are kept. These reactions are not only visible in instances where markers have been included intentionally, they are also an indicator of the individual's comprehension of natural markers in daily routines.

In order for the individual to understand the significance of the markers, it is of vital importance that they are presented immediately prior to the activities. If too much time passes between the marker being presented and the activity taking place, distracting events may interfere and make it difficult for the individual to understand the relationship between the markers and the activities they signal.

> Hannah is a mentally handicapped girl of 7. She is led by the hand to feel her bathing costume as a signal that she is going swim-

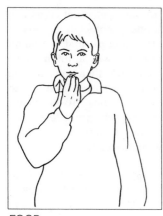

FOOD

ming. She is then dressed, led to the bus stop, waits 15 minutes for the bus, sits on the bus for 20 minutes, walks for 5 minutes, goes to the changing room, undresses, puts on her bathing costume and finally goes swimming.

Using markers in the manner indicated above is unsuitable in the early stages of teaching. It can be difficult to understand that the bathing costume signals a visit to the swimming pool, not one of the activities that always occurs beforehand.

When teaching the significance of markers it is also important that they are not presented at too late a stage. For example, it is not very appropriate to use the sign FOOD to inform individuals that they are going to eat when they are already seated at the table. The sign is superfluous, and thus meaningless, because it does not signal a change in the situation. The fact that they are going to eat has already been conveyed through a large number of natural markers: the food is on the table, there is a smell of food, they are wearing bibs, etc. The sign should be performed before they enter the dining room or, at the very least, before they are seated at the table.

Once the signal sign has been learned, the interval between the presentation of the sign and the situation should gradually be lengthened, so that it becomes possible to talk about activities that will not take place immediately. This will also lay the foundation for individuals to either ask for things that are not visible or express a wish to participate in activities that are not taking place at the time of asking.

Marker-controlled frame structuring may be combined with the use of a timetable with pictures or PIC signs or a day box with rows containing objects, as is common in structured total communication. However, the markers and the fixed order of the various activities are the crucial elements in the teaching. These must be understood in the context of the particular situation before they can be presented independently of it. Reviewing the day's markers before the individuals can clearly demonstrate an understanding of what the markers signal may make it more difficult for them to learn the signal function of these markers.

The use of markers in order to provide individuals with a better understanding of their own environment is not dependent on frame structuring. Signal signs and other markers may be used to sign activities and events even though the events do not occur daily or at the same time every day. They may be used with all activities and events that are repeated sufficiently often enough for it to be a reasonable assumption that the individuals will be able to understand the signs. Using signal signs in daily routines or in other situations where the same activities or events occur in the same order is especially useful because the fixed order and use of signal signs have a mutually enhancing effect. The signal signs facilitate the individuals' understanding of the situation, and an understanding of the situation facilitates their understanding of the signs.

In environments where use and comprehension of manual signs are taught it is usual for signal signs also to be used outside the planned situations. This is more unusual when graphic signs are used. The graphic signs should be used so that the individuals have the chance to learn from non-planned comprehension experiences, if they are able to do so. In cases where the individuals need to learn that a sign corresponds to a specific word, the graphic signs should be used in conjunction with speech whenever this is practical. In this way the individuals' comprehension (and possibly use) of the sign and the word may be associated with several situations. For people with a poor understanding of language, the simultaneous use of signs and speech may also make it easier for them to understand the words that are being spoken.

Special training

Comprehension training in special teaching situations can be classified according to the person performing the sign – the individual or the teacher. When teaching manual sign comprehension the teacher generally displays a picture or points at an object, and the person has to perform the manual sign that corresponds to that picture or object. When teaching graphic sign comprehension the individual has to point at the graphic sign. This is the equivalent of naming. However, the most common form of comprehension training is for the teacher to perform the manual sign or point at the graphic sign. The learner then has to point to the corresponding object or picture, pick it up, or perform an activity. The teacher points at the graphic sign or performs a manual sign, and simultaneously says the word that corresponds to the sign. In this type of comprehension training the individual generally has to choose among several objects or pictures. The positioning of the pictures or objects should vary, so that the individual does not merely learn to pick up the object or point at the picture that occupies one particular position.

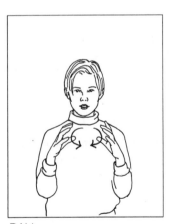

BALL

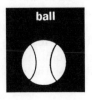

> Dan is a 15-year-old mentally handicapped boy. A ball and a spoon are placed in front of him on a table. The teacher says 'ball' while performing the sign BALL. Dan gives the ball to the teacher (Booth, 1978).

Comprehension training in which the teacher uses the signs and the individual points at an object is less common in graphic sign teaching than it is in manual sign teaching. This is partly because the manual sign must be performed each time it is used, while the graphic sign is present the whole time. The teacher becomes used to performing manual signs, but not to pointing at graphic signs. The main reason, however, is probably that because many graphic signs are stylised drawings, the teacher seems to assume the individual will understand them immediately.

As there appears – with the exception of signal signs – to be no tradition of teaching graphic sign comprehension, this is probably related to the fact that the Bliss system was the first sign system to be adopted. Many of the first individuals to be taught in the use of graphic signs had a good understanding of language (cf. Vanderheiden et al., 1975). For people who belong to this group, comprehension training is the equivalent of rote learning whereby the individual learns that a sign corresponds to a specific word. The most simple and effective way of teaching sign comprehension is for the teacher to say the words without having to find objects or pictures that the sign may be used to describe. Comprehension training, where the learner has to pick up or touch objects or point at pictures, is best suited for individuals belonging to the alternative language group and the supportive language group. For those who belong to the expressive language group and who have a good understanding of language, a more appropriate approach is first to explain in words the signs that are to be learned, and then perhaps check how well the signs are remembered by asking the individual to translate the words that the teacher has said into graphic or manual signs.

Teaching sign use

There are many ways of training people in the use of signs, and they may be classified in different ways. Most of them may be used in special training and natural environments.

Watch—Wait—React

The purpose of this strategy is to transform into signs casual activity produced by the individual, by reacting as though that activity was communicative. Reactions of this kind are similar to the *over-interpretation* found among the parents of children who develop language normally. The teaching may take place in unstructured situations, and nothing special need be done to encourage specific activities. The individual is observed – watched. As soon as a movement is made that may be recognised if repeated at a later stage, the teacher reacts to this movement as though the individual had performed a specific sign. This method is best suited for individuals with a low degree of self-initiated activity.

This strategy may have several positive effects. For example, there is reason to believe that the passivity that often characterises children with poor language and communication skills is related to the fact that they display behaviour that elicits reaction from others to a lesser degree than other children do (Ryan, 1977). The strategy of Watch – Wait – React increases the chances of an individual's activities eliciting a reaction, which will probably stimulate the level of activity and initiative to communicate. The object of this strategy is that the teacher's reactions to the individual's casual activity should have a spiralling effect, with the reactions causing new activities on the part of the individual. This will improve the learning opportunities for individuals with severely impaired communication skills. The new activities may then in turn be ascribed a similar sign function. In this way a positive spiral of development is started. For this to happen, it is best that the activities to which the teacher reacts are, to begin with, expressions of the individual's awareness and motivation. This will also increase the likelihood of the individual becoming aware of the relationship between what is happening in the situation, his or her own activities, and the reactions of people in the surroundings.

> Harold is a 4-year-old mentally handicapped boy. He is passive and shows very little self-initiated activity. He likes to be lifted up and played with roughly. Sometimes he beats his breast. This is 'interpreted' by his parents and the nursery school staff as 'I want to play', and each time he beats his breast, he is lifted up and played with.

The Watch – Wait – React strategy has clear limitations. The person who administers the teaching has very little control over when a selected casual activity will occur, and can run the risk of having to wait for a long time before it is repeated. It is crucial that the individual is attentive and that the reactions manage to catch the individual's interest. One may secure these conditions to a certain extent by beginning with an activity that occurs relatively often and basing the sign's 'content' on information about the learner's interests.

Reacting to habitual behaviour

This strategy is most suitable for individuals who have some degree of self-initiated activity, although that activity is not

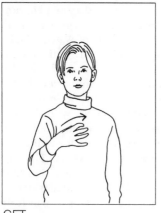

GET

functional. For example, reacting to habitual behaviour is a strategy that suits children and adults who, when left to their own devices, wander aimlessly around a room, kick walls and furniture, hit a table if they pass one by, or pull objects down from shelves. The strategy is based on knowing what the individual will do in a given situation, and what he or she will be interested in. The object is to make a non-functional activity communicative and socially acceptable. In order to achieve this, one must produce a teaching situation in which it is possible to trigger off the activity and utilise it for sign teaching.

> Andrew is an 8-year-old autistic boy. He has a tendency to empty any handbags he can get his hands on. He is placed in a room in which a person is sitting with a handbag, and where nothing special is happening. The teacher follows him as he walks around the room. As soon as he reaches for the bag, he is held back by his teacher who forms the sign HANDBAG with his hands. He is then given the bag by the person who is sitting there.

Alternatively, Andrew could have been taught to use a general sign such as GET or GIVE, depending on what the teacher felt was most useful.

The purpose of this strategy is to give habitual behaviour that has previously been non-functional a sign function by systematically reacting to the behaviour as though it was communicative. This strategy is based on the learner identifying his or her own activity with the reaction on the part of the conversational partner. For the strategy to succeed, it is essential that the individual's attention is captured by both his or her own behaviour and the reaction of the teacher, so that he or she will want the reaction to be repeated.

One advantage of the strategy of reacting to habitual behaviour is that what is generally regarded as problematic behaviour may be taken as a starting point and exploited to the individual's advantage. Since the behaviour is replaced by a sign and is given a positive function, it may be said that the sign teaching has simultaneously led to an unlearning of the problematic behaviour. Another advantage is that the teacher is able to decide on the timing of the training in advance by planning a situation in which the behaviour occurs habitually. This provides the teacher with control over the sign teaching which, among other things, will ensure a sufficient number of repetitions.

Build-and-break chains

This strategy is based on constructing a chain of activities that the individual is motivated to carry out, and then obstructing the chain so that it is impossible to complete it

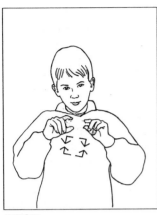

PIECE

without help. When the individual shows frustration, he or she is guided to produce a manual sign or point at a graphic sign. The teacher then sees to it that the individual is given the chance of continuing the chain of behaviour. This strategy can be utilised among individuals with varying levels of activity, and is especially suitable for people who need to learn to do things on their own initiative.

Both learned activity chains and naturally occurring chains (routines) may be used as basis for the Build-and-break chain strategy, providing that the individual is sufficiently well motivated in the situation. The chains need not be long.

> Carl is a 10-year-old autistic boy. He has learned to complete a simple jigsaw puzzle where the pieces are placed from left to right. Carl has learned to take the correct piece of puzzle. The chain is broken by pushing the pieces out of his reach, so that Carl needs help to get hold of them. There are two teachers. One sits behind Carl and helps, while the other sits in front of him and tends to the pieces. As soon as Carl discovers he is missing one of the pieces of the jigsaw puzzle (preferably not the first piece), he reaches for it without getting hold of it and looks at the teacher sitting in front of him. The helper guides his hands to perform the sign PIECE. Then the other teacher gives him the piece of jigsaw puzzle he needs.

It is essential that the individual is motivated to carry out the chain before it is broken for the purpose of sign teaching. This is not always an easy task. One way of ensuring the individual's motivation is to begin by breaking the chain when the last link in the chain precedes something that the individual wishes to do. For example, for someone who is fond of going for a drive, the fixed routine of getting dressed before going for a drive can be interrupted. Sometimes humour and surprise can be used to break the chain.

The Build-and-break chain strategy involves frustrating the learner. Frustration works because a need for communication arises and makes it clear to the individual that using signs can be expedient. It is vital that the frustration the individual is subjected to – in the eyes of the learner – appears to be the result of situational circumstances; it should not appear to be produced by the conversational partner, who should act as a helper.

Reacting to marker-triggered anticipatory behaviour

The strategy of reacting to marker-triggered anticipatory behaviour assumes that the teacher has constructed a frame structure in which known activities or events occur in a specific order, and where the activities or events have a precur-

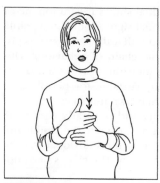

WORK

sory marker. When the individuals begin to demonstrate that they understand what is going to happen, the anticipatory reaction they show may be used in the sign teaching. If the anticipatory reaction is appropriate, it may be used as a sign, or their hands can be guided to form a sign immediately after the anticipatory reaction.

The strategy assumes that the activity or event the individuals have anticipated will follow naturally once the individuals have reacted. In practical terms this means that a chain is produced by placing a sign between the links. The chain will end with the activity the marker indicates.

> Elaine is a 19-year-old autistic girl. She enjoys basket-weaving. This activity is indicated by the sign WORK. She is well acquainted with this situation and looks in the direction of the shelf where the basket-weaving materials are kept when the teacher says and signs WORK. As Elaine looks towards the shelf, her hands are formed to make the sign MATERIAL and the materials are then fetched.

This is one example of the use of frame structure, where a comprehension sign is used as a marker for a group of activities. These may be various activities pertaining to work or sports, which are often suitable for producing a situation in which the individuals will gradually learn to choose between different activities with the help of signs.

If the individuals display marker-triggered anticipatory behaviour, then several of the basic conditions that are essential to the success of the teaching are already present. The individuals are attentive, motivated and have an understanding of what the situation entails. This makes it easier for them to learn to understand and begin using the sign. In addition, the teacher has control over what is going to happen in advance, and is able to use the structuring as a tool with which to encourage activity in individuals whose behavioural repertoire is limited.

Fulfilling wants

This is the most commonly used strategy. It may be used in both natural and special training situations, and is a strategy that may be used with all the three main groups. For the supportive language and alternative language groups, it is an instrument with which to teach individuals that they can achieve something by using language. For the expressive language group, the strategy is expedient for unlearning learned helplessness, and showing individuals that they can achieve a particular goal by using signs. The same strategy can thus have different objectives.

When fulfilling the desire of individuals to carry out a particular activity, their likes and interests should be borne

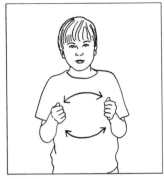

CAR

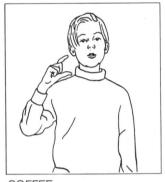

COFFEE

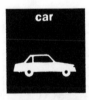

in mind and used as a starting point. The teacher should create a situation that makes the individuals want to carry out the activity, mould their hands to make the manual sign or point at the graphic sign, and then let them perform the activity they want. Similarly, the teacher fulfils an individual's wish for a particular thing by using an object he or she knows that person wants. This may be something the individual likes to do something with or play with, something to eat or drink, etc. The teacher waits until the individual shows in one way or another that the particular object is wanted, guides his or her hands to form the sign or point at a graphic sign, and then provides the object.

Henry is a 7-year-old autistic boy. He likes to crank the ladder on his toy fire-engine up and down. The teacher walks together with Henry and makes sure that they pass the fire-engine. When Henry clearly looks at the fire-engine, stops or reaches for it, the teacher moulds his hands to perform the sign CAR, whereupon Henry is given the fire-engine.

Elaine is a 43-year old multiply handicapped woman, who is dependent on a wheelchair. She is fond of coffee, which she drinks with a straw, but she herself never takes the initiative to get coffee. She can press the keys on a talking aid with digitised speech. The teacher has recorded the word coffee on her talking aid and places the PIC sign COFFEE on the key that she presses. The teacher sits close by Elaine with two cups and a coffee pot. When Elaine looks at the teacher, she approaches her and helps Elaine to press the key with the sign COFFEE. The machine says coffee and the teacher pours Elaine a cup.

Although individuals who are taught manual or graphic signs generally perform few activities and appear to like few things, this is not the only reason why these same things and activities are repeated. Those who plan the teaching often show too little imagination and creativity. There are, after all, many areas from which to chose. There are toys and games, household objects, food, sweets, fruit, clothes and shoes, cassette players, television and radio, cuddling, gymnastics, outdoor activities, etc. A craft session may include DRAW, PAPER, CUT and GLUE. Physical activity may be DANCE. Looking at a MAGAZINE is enjoyable. In northern Norway, for example, REINDEER is a useful animal. It is also easy to overlook the fact that preferences and interests change as the individual becomes older and learns new skills.

Sometimes the objects indicated by the signs the individuals are being taught are easily available in the environment. An open shelf located high up on the wall may be practical. Since the shelf is open, any objects placed there are visible, which may help the individuals to remember them and want to get hold of them. Since the shelf is

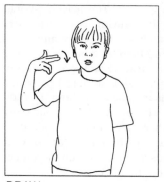

DRAW

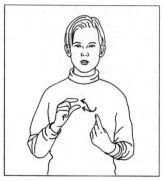

PAPER

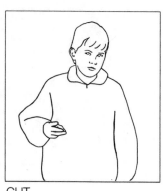

CUT

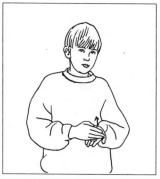

GLUE

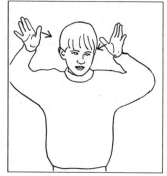

REINDEER

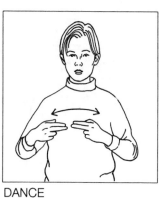

DANCE

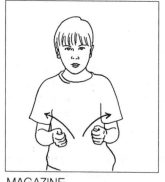

MAGAZINE

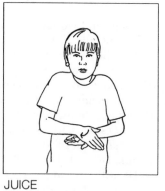

JUICE

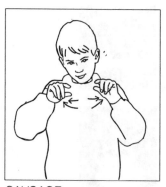

SAUSAGE

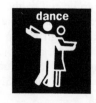

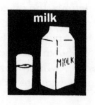

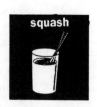

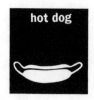

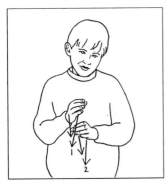

MILK

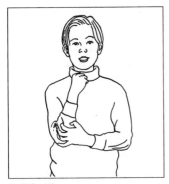

BISCUIT

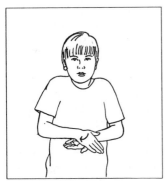

JUICE/SQUASH

placed high up on the wall, the individuals are unable to reach the object unaided, and this provides them with the opportunity of approaching another person for help.

Signs for food and drink are often chosen as early object signs because it is generally known what the people like to eat and drink. Signs such as MILK, BISCUITS, SQUASH and SAUSAGE are also easy to administer during the teaching. However, it may not always be advisable to start teaching food signs at meal times. It is easy to take away from individuals communication skills that they already possess and ruin a pleasant situation at the same time. Instead, the sign training can be carried out in the place where the meals are usually served, but a short while before the meal begins. Once the signs are mastered in this situation, they can be introduced carefully during meal times. One way to do this is to 'forget' to put something the individual likes on the table, and use this ploy to teach that signs can be a tool for getting something that is not there, and thereby a means of improving a situation.

It is essential that sign use does not become a ritual, but that it actually leads to an improved situation for the individual. Although the signs for food or drink are often well suited to the first stages of sign teaching, they are occasionally unsuitable because they do not lead to increased functional communication. If a boy already has a means of expressing clearly to the people around him that he wants orange juice, by smacking his lips for example, and expects to be given orange juice when he does so, the purpose of using a sign to achieve the same thing may be unclear to him. He would have to be taught not to smack his lips before he could be taught to use the sign JUICE. In such instances, learning signs to express things the individual is already capable of communicating in other ways may lead to a confusion about their purpose, and it is more expedient to begin with teaching other signs.

Some physically disabled children have difficulty chewing and swallowing, and eating is therefore an activity they do reluctantly. In such cases choosing between different types of food is not a suitable strategy to use. On the other hand, it can be advantageous for the individual to achieve improved control over meals in terms of choosing when the next bite of food will be consumed and when he or she wishes to drink (Morris, 1981).

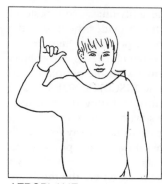

AEROPLANE

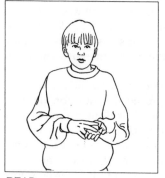

READ

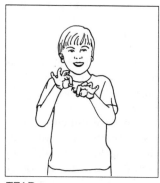

TEAR

Incidental Teaching

Incidental teaching is the term used to describe a situation where the teaching or subject matter has not been decided upon in advance. However, this does not mean that the situation is not planned. The teacher may know that the individual is interested in a specific activity and has planned that he should learn the sign for this activity, without setting a time for when the teaching should take place. Sometimes incidental teaching can take place without the teacher knowing what the individual is interested in. If a situation is created in which it is likely that the individual will want something, and the teacher then waits for the expression of interest in an unstructured situation, the incidental teaching corresponds to the Watch—Wait—React strategy.

> Eric is a 6-year-old autistic boy. He stands in front of a cupboard and performs all the manual signs he knows. When the cupboard is opened he reaches out for a model aeroplane in the cupboard. His hand is quickly guided to make the sign AEROPLANE, and Eric is given the aeroplane.

> Claire is a 12-year-old mentally handicapped girl. She holds a book in her hand and stands looking at her teacher. Her hand is guided to make the sign READ. Claire is then allowed to sit on the teacher's lap while the teacher reads for her.

> Betty is an 8-year-old multiply handicapped girl. She sits in a wheelchair. During morning assembly at nursery school she looks intently at the pages of the large calendar that one of the children is allowed to tear off. The assistant fetches the PIC sign TEAR, puts it together with the other PIC signs on the tray attached to the wheelchair and guides Betty to point to it. The calendar is taken to Betty and, with help from the assistant, she tears off the page.

The advantages of incidental teaching are that it provides more teaching situations, and that the teaching takes place in situations where the individual is motivated and has a use for the sign. Incidental teaching may be used with both new signs and signs that are being practised, depending on the situation. However, this is conditional on the signs being easily accessible, i.e. that the person in charge of the incidental teaching knows the required manual signs, and that the graphic signs are available in all situations.

Professionals often have reservations about teaching signs that are not a part of the planned programme. They are afraid that the situation will be too difficult for the individuals to grasp, and that they may find it confusing. The teacher's own knowledge of manual signs or the graphic system used may also be a limitation, although this is not usually the cause of the problem. It does not take very long to teach someone a few new manual signs or set out a number of graphic signs so that they are easily accessible.

aeroplane

read

tear

There are also examples of instances where the learning of new signs has stopped, and where the effect of the introduction of incidental teaching has been similar to that of a tap being turned on. The reason for this *may* be that the sign teaching has taken place in too restricted a situation, so that the individual has not understood the difference between signs, but that the incidental teaching created sufficient situational variation. It may also be the case that the teaching situation itself had become monotonous and ritualistic, and thus no longer contributed to the learning of new signs.

This presentation of incidental teaching differs in part from the descriptions that are given in a number of other contexts (Carr, 1985; Oliver and Halle, 1982). The main difference is that for us incidental teaching has as its aim that *the communication should be successful*. In much of the literature incidental teaching is regarded as *an opportunity to establish a teaching situation*. Despite the fact that the teaching begins on a communicative initiative from the individual, the linguistic aims are decided upon in advance (Warren and Kaiser, 1986). The teacher also uses methods employed in special training, i.e. the use of prompting, imitation, etc., and thus interrupts the communication.

Structured waiting

As a way of making life easier for disabled people, many parents and professionals anticipate their needs and give them what they require. This implies at the same time that they remove one aspect of the situation that makes communication useful. The result may be that the individuals are not given the opportunity of taking the initiative in situations where this would otherwise have been natural. This creates a form of learned passivity. In order to increase the chances that the individuals themselves will initiate communication, structured waiting can be introduced in natural teaching situations or on occasions in incidental teaching when one believes that an individual will use a *known* sign. This implies waiting for a short space of time before prompts are made or help given to perform a sign. It is usual to begin with a very short interval and gradually increase the time to approximately 10 seconds. It is possible to wait even longer, but it appears that longer periods of waiting seldom lead to self-initiation among people without motor impairments (Oliver and Halle, 1982). Among motor-impaired individuals who have difficulty in pointing or performing manual signs, it may be necessary to wait longer (cf. Light, 1985).

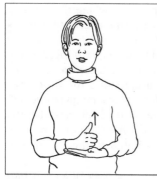

HELP

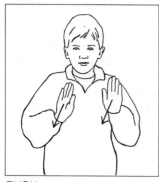

PUSH

Jay is a 7-year-old boy with a motor impairment. He was taken to the changing room to change clothes before exercising. He needed help with the button on his trousers. The teacher held her finger on the button but waited 10 seconds before Jay, on the occasions he needed it, was given help in performing the sign HELP.

Jay used to push a scooter together with his physiotherapist as a means of training his arm muscles. The physiotherapist stopped and waited for 10 seconds for Jay to perform the sign PUSH before she would help Jay to perform the sign (Oliver and Halle, 1982).

By waiting, the chances that individuals will take the initiative in a communicative situation are increased. Doing so will make them more active and break down learned passivity. It has also been shown that the time it takes to learn new signs will be reduced if postponed help is included as part of the teaching strategy (Bennet et al., 1986).

Structured waiting can be very important for people with motor impairments who belong to the expressive language group. The motor impairment means that they spend longer both answering and taking the initiative. If they are to be more than just responsive, and be able to take more initiative, the conversational partner must give them sufficient time. Mentally handicapped people who belong to one of the other main groups can also be slow and take time responding and showing initiative. Thus, structured waiting has a double function. It creates a need for communication and places restrictions on the conversational partners, so that they become more aware that they should not give help unless it is absolutely necessary. Intentional postponement of help may be used even with small children (cf. Light, 1985).

Naming

Naming contains elements of both comprehension and use. Giving names to objects and events is a normal linguistic activity, which is found in the very early stages of language acquisition, often in situations where children and their parents look at books or toys together. In augmentative communication, naming is used to teach the individual the name of objects and pictures, not to use them. The teaching generally takes place in special teaching situations. It is the learners who have to point at the graphic sign or perform the manual sign. The individuals do not learn to use the manual sign or graphic sign in new ways, they learn only to answer questions when the object is present or a picture of an object or an event is shown.

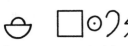

?

what

bag   television

telephone

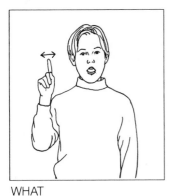

WHAT

Peter is 4 years old. He has a motor impairment but shows good language comprehension. He sits together with his teacher at his nursery school. She has different objects around her and points at an object or a picture of a particular object while simultaneously pronouncing the word that corresponds to the sign. Peter points at the Blissymbols on his board as the teacher says the words.

Kate is an autistic girl of 14. She uses a number of signs and a few words. She sits with her teacher, who points at various objects and says 'What is that?' while performing the sign WHAT. Kate then performs the appropriate manual sign, and is given help where necessary.

Naming can be an appropriate way of learning new names, but requires that individuals have learned to use a number of signs in order to obtain objects and participate in activities. It is useful to be able to answer questions, but this is not a goal of the preliminary teaching. For children and adults with good language skills who are thought to be capable of translating their comprehension into functional use, naming is a good method of acquiring new signs.

Structured and unstructured situations

Structuring of the teaching situation is one of the best tools available in language and communication training. In particular, conscious structuring is a suitable tool in the teaching of individuals with the poorest qualifications for language acquisition. The less self-initiated activity an individual has, the greater the need for a rigid structuring. A rigid structuring represents the best way of achieving more self-initiated activity among low-functioning individuals and breaking up their life of passivity. Another objective is that also people with extensive disabilities should achieve the greatest possible control over what happens to them, and should be able to take the initiative in everyday life and choose what they themselves want to do. The easiest way to achieve this is to create a structured teaching situation.

It has been claimed that structuring an environment and fostering individual initiative and choice are mutually contradictory but, in our opinion, this is not so. On the contrary, planned use of structuring can increase the level of activity and provide individuals with a basis for gaining greater freedom of choice. Several of the strategies employed in expressive teaching utilise structuring to foster communication and initiative. The Build-and-break strategy utilises the situational structure in order to create a need for communication. Reactions to marker-triggered anticipatory behaviour use the frame structure in a similar way. Frame structuring is also suited to the task of establishing choice between activities.

Although structuring is one of the most useful tools available for developing situational understanding and communication, it is also important to be aware that structure is a *help condition* and not a goal in itself. Most people have a relatively structured existence. They get up in the morning, eat breakfast, go to school or work, eat dinner, watch television, etc. However, the structure is fairly flexible; watching television may be replaced by a trip to the cinema, an evening playing bridge, a social gathering with friends, etc. A correspondingly flexible structure is the ideal objective for people who receive structured teaching. Thus, the aim of structuring is to form the basis of the development of flexible behavioural patterns and the ability to make decisions. This means that the structure is changed as soon as there is a basis for doing so.

Once a successful frame structure has been established, i.e. when the day's activities seem to be understood and are carried out well enough, it is probably time to begin dismantling the structure. In many cases the situations for the individuals concerned may be so structured, have taken place with virtually no complications, and have remained unchanged for such a long period of time, that there is no natural need for communication in their daily routines. The markers have become rituals, and no longer help to build up new understanding about the environment. The individual may be so tied to the frame structure and the markers that these now preclude the development of new skills and choices instead of strengthening this development. This may be called *learned dependence*.

After an over-ritualised structure has been dismantled, the individuals may still have a need for a *time aid*. Such an aid may be a calendar that helps individuals to understand the differences between the days; weekdays and public holidays, vacations and working days.

Edward is an 18-year-old autistic boy who understands a little speech. When his daily routine was broken up by holidays he had violent temper tantrums. It was difficult to quieten him down and he had to be held so that he did not hurt himself or others. Edward's mother drew a calendar for him on which were included the things she knew he liked (Figure 28). To represent the days he spent at school, she drew a picture of a bus since he always looked forward to taking the bus. On some of his days off from school he is allowed to drive his uncle's tractor. On Saturday they always mop the floor. On Sundays he has egg for breakfast. Christmas shopping, the Christmas holidays and New Year's Eve are all represented with drawings that are easy to understand. The calendar hangs in one place in the kitchen. Every morning Edward looks at it to find out what that particular day will bring. Each evening he crosses off the day that has passed. Since Edward was given the calendar, his holidays have been much more peace-

Figure 28. *Calendar of an 18-year-old autistic boy.*

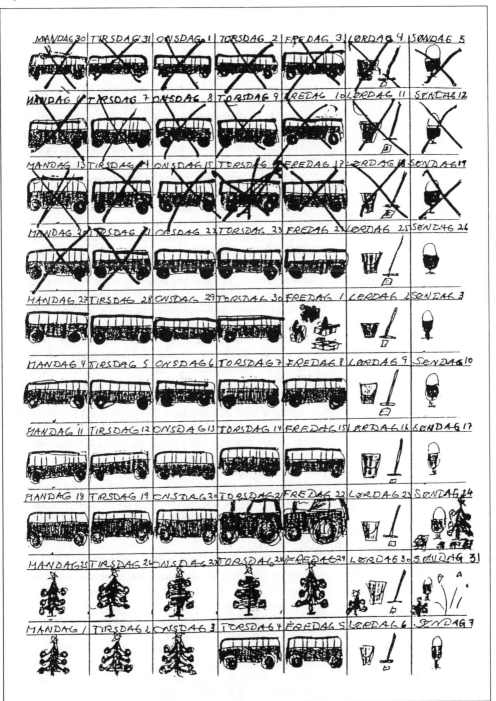

ful. It appears as though it was important for him to know that he was going back to school, and that this part of his life was not over even though the holidays were long (K. Steindal, personal communication 1990).

Preparatory training

Language and communication teaching often begins with the learning of skills, knowledge or activities that are regarded as conditions for language acquisition. It is often a stated requirement that these conditions must be present before the language teaching commences. One example of this is the requirement that the child 'be in possession of' concepts that correspond to the words before these can be learned, which is based on the theory that concepts must exist before language. Other examples are the requirements that the child has concepts of amount or object constancy (Chapman and Miller, 1980; Shane and Bashir, 1981). The ability to imitate has also been regarded as a necessary precursor to language acquisition (Piaget and Inhelder, 1969; Skinner, 1957). The assumption that such fundamental preconditions must exist in order for the child to acquire language has little empirical basis, however, and has often led to inefficient teaching and hindered the acquisition of communication. There are many examples of individuals who have not reached Piaget's sensory-motor stage V or VI, but who have nonetheless been able to use language (Bonvillian, Orlansky and Novack, 1981; Reichle and Karlan, 1985).

Another type of condition that is stressed has to do with the practical implementation of language teaching. Some skills or activities are regarded as necessary, or extremely advantageous, if language teaching is to be effective. One example of such a skill is being able to sit still on a chair in front of a table for a certain period of time. Other examples are the ability to be attentive and look at the teacher. Motivation to communicate has also been emphasised as a practical condition (cf. Bryen and Joyce, 1985; Vanderheiden et al., 1975).

Teaching the individual skills and activities that may contribute to a more effective language teaching at a later stage is positive, and in line with the necessity of regarding different interventionary measures in a wider perspective. But this teaching should not be at the expense of communication teaching. Such skills and activities are a part of the total intervention and not a necessary requirement for the commencement of communication teaching. Teaching of such skills should take place concurrently with the language teaching and will thus not lead to a loss of time.

There are a number of theoretical and practical conditions that have been given special attention. These include *eye contact, direction of gaze, attentiveness, sitting still, behaviour chains, imitation* and *motor skills.*

Eye contact

In many interventionary measures involving autistic people the establishment of eye contact has been of major importance, and eye contact has often been an important aim before the implementation of language teaching. This is because the lack of eye contact has been regarded as a sign of a contact disorder. However, there is no support for the theory that the establishment of eye contact is a necessary precondition for language acquisition. In addition, it is difficult to look another person in the eyes and simultaneously look at one's own or others' signs.

Direction of gaze and attentiveness

In particular, individuals with autism and mental retardation have been given training in the direction of gaze and attentiveness, but the expressive language group has also been trained to aim its gaze at objects before they have begun to use graphic sign systems.

There are two different argument that form the justification for the special emphasis on training the direction of gaze. The first justification is that intended communication is essential to the learning of language because it precedes words in normal development. A change in the direction of gaze, i.e. the child looking alternately at an object and the adult helper, has been used as a measure of intended communication (Bates, 1979). Training the direction of gaze has thus been regarded as training in intended communication.

The second justification is more practical. The direction of gaze is regarded as an expression of attentiveness, and training in directing one's gaze at a person or thing is a form of attentiveness training.

Attentiveness is a fundamental prerequisite for the success of language teaching, and initiating contact with another person may be a prerequisite for the use of a sign to be perceived as communication. For example, autistic individuals often look away from the direction in which they are pointing and the pointing is therefore not considered communicative. Many people with extensive motor impairments are not perceived as communicating because the listener does not notice that they are attentive. They may not have the ability to hold their head up, change the direction of gaze, etc. However, practising these skills in advance is not particularly productive. An understanding of how to initiate contact and get the attention of another person can only be expected to be understood in a functional context. Similarly, it can be futile to train individuals to direct their gaze at another person unless it is clear why this has a purpose. Reinforcing such behaviour, by giving sweets for example, only causes greater confusion. Both attentiveness and the initiation of contact are easier to bring out in an actual communicative situation than by special training.

Looking at the object that forms the basis of the communication will often be a part of the actual sign teaching, for example by the teacher using this as a first indicator of the individual's choice or attentiveness. In turn this is a basis for helping the individual form the sign. In the teaching of aided communication using eye pointing, the direction of gaze is the actual communicative expression and will then be learned in a functional communicative context.

Sitting still

The requirement that an individual sits still at a table for a certain length of time is very commonplace in the teaching of augmentative communication. As a rule mentally handicapped and autistic individuals have been taught to sit still, but so to some extent have restless children with less extensive disorders belonging to the supportive language group.

It can be expedient to teach the individual to sit still at a table because it facilitates the performance of a large number of activities that are generally performed at a table; painting, building with Lego bricks, doing jigsaw puzzles, etc. Such activities have their own value and may also be utilised in communication teaching. Training in sitting still is thus justified not on the grounds of communication teaching, but rather because of the objective that the individuals take part in activities that are performed at a table. If one teaches individuals to sit still, by using, for example, the command signs SIT and STILL, and then make them unlearn this so that they can carry out an activity (point at or perform a sign), this necessitates a good deal of extra work and loss of time. At the beginning of the communication teaching, the individuals may be anxious and unsettled because the situation is new, they have very little grasp of what is going on and do not know what demands will be made on them. As they gradually become familiar with the situation they will have expectations of that situation and understand what is expected of them. Their anxiety will then disappear (Schaeffer, Musil and Kollinzas, 1980).

Restlessness can also be an expression of an interest that may be utilised in the teaching.

Tracy is a 6-year-old autistic girl. Her chief interest was running in the corridors at school. The first thing she learned was therefore the manual sign RUN. When she ran towards the door in order to run out into the corridor, she was stopped and guided to make the manual sign before she left the room. There were many chances to repeat this, and the sign was used spontaneously from the very first day. The teaching continued in the gymnasium with the signs JUMP and CLIMB (K. Steindal, personal communication 1990).

Behaviour chains

Skills and activities that give one something to talk about are fundamental to all language teaching. When starting language teaching for autistic or mentally handicapped people, the teacher may often find that they possess few such skills and activities. This may mean that they need to be taught behaviour chains, i.e. that several activities must be performed consecutively. A simple behavioural chain might consist of fetching building bricks and building a small tower. Learning to ride a bicycle involves a chain of advanced motor skills.

The development of behaviour chains will take place at the same time as language teaching, often with the use of signal signs. The primary purpose of building behaviour chains is to improve individuals' independence and under-standing of their own environment, but the behaviour chains may also be used in language teaching. In the case of extremely low-functioning individuals, not all behaviour

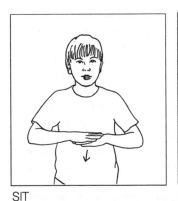
SIT

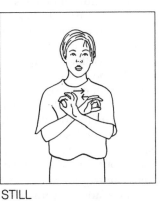
STILL

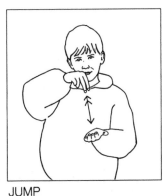
JUMP

sit

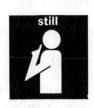
still

jump

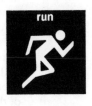
run

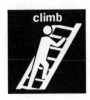
climb

chains will be identified with graphic or manual signs, and behaviour chains that are established without signs can be practical to use when the sign teaching is expanded.

Imitation

Imitation training has been argued for both as a prerequisite for other learning and as a skill that is functional in itself. Imitation as a necessary prerequisite for learning has led to an emphasis on training of imitation as a 'metaskill', i.e. a general ability to follow the instruction: *Do as I do*. This type of metaskill usually appears late in development, however, and the first things children imitate are *skills they have already mastered*. Children who are only 1 year old can imitate someone combing themselves with a comb, but will refuse to comb themselves with a toy car. Even children who are a good deal older can appear fairly frustrated if they are asked to do the same as, for example, someone who places her hand on her head (Guillaume, 1971). This implies that the imitation is an unsuitable strategy for teaching new skills in early development.

In the preliminary stages of imitation training, the children are often given help in performing the action they have to imitate. When a child is later able to imitate the action this may be taken as an indicator that the *action* has been learned, rather than that the imitation has been learned as a general principle. So although the imitation training appears to have been successful, in the sense that the individual imitates specific activities or sounds, this does not necessarily mean that the skill will be generalised, i.e. that an individual will more easily begin to imitate signs or words that other people are using.

The fact that imitation is not a prerequisite for language acquisition has been fully demonstrated by children and adults with extensive motor impairments. Many individuals who are barely able to imitate any action nonetheless develop the ability to solve problems, good language comprehension and use of language through writing or graphic signs. Also, severely mentally handicapped people who have not been taught imitation have learned to use graphic and manual signs.

There are few studies that have compared imitation and hand guidance in sign teaching. Iacono and Parsons (1986) used these two teaching strategies in the teaching of three severely mentally handicapped youths between the ages of 11 and 15. Two of them had never been taught manual signs. The third adolescent had been taught to use the sign DRINK several years earlier, but had never used the sign spontaneously. In an evaluation of their imitation skills, one of the youths (F.L.) managed to imitate 6 out of 10 gestures,

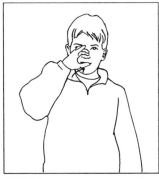

DRINK

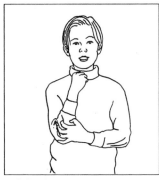

BISCUIT

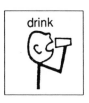

while the other two did not manage to imitate any of them.

The teaching was designed so that the manual signs BISCUIT and DRINK or BISCUIT and LOLLIPOP were first attempted to be taught with the aid of imitation. Then an attempt was made to teach one sign using imitation, and the other using hand guidance. Finally, both the signs were taught using hand guidance. The results demonstrated clearly that imitation was not a good teaching strategy for these individuals (Figure 29). Even F.L., who had managed to imitate gestures, was unable to benefit from the imitation training.

The necessity of being able to imitate on practical grounds is to a large extent a legacy from traditional speech training, where imitating sounds is a major element. It is extremely difficult to carry out speech training without the imitation of sounds, because it is not easy to manipulate the lips, tongue and other parts of an individual's articulatory organs in order to get him or her to pronounce a specific word. One of the great advantages of augmentative communication is that imitation is not necessary, because help and guidance in pointing at and performing signs can be given in other ways. Imitation *can* be a useful strategy, but on the condition that the individual has an understanding of what the imitation is about, i.e. imitation has been acquired as a metaskill.

Motor skills

Preparatory motor training has been given particular emphasis in the teaching of individuals with motor disorders. Certain motor skills are necessary in order to be able to use a communication aid, but often the mastering of one specific way of use forms the basis for whether the individual will be allowed to use an aid. Although, as a rule, individuals have most motor control over the head, it is usual to teach them first to use their hands to activate switches.

The training of the motor skills that are needed to use a communication aid should take place at the same time as the teaching in the use of the aid. This can be done by allowing the individuals to play a game, carry out environmental control, or perform other activities that utilise the same movement. At the same time the sign system can be used in a dependent way so that the individual becomes acquainted with it. For example, if an individual is given a communication aid that utilises automatic scanning, it can be used at first with dependent scanning, in which the conversational partner points and the person indicates when he or she is pointing at the right column and word. Subsequently, the individual learns to master independent scanning.

Figure 29. *Learning curves of imitation and guidance (Iacono and Parsons, 1986). The lowest possible score is 60, the highest is 20.*

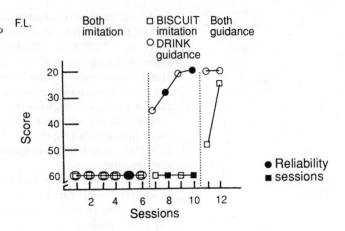

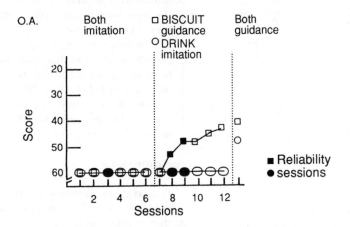

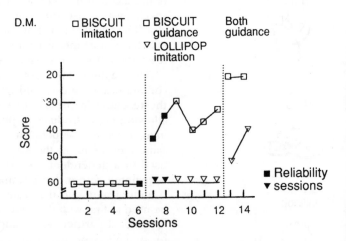

Chapter 8
Choosing the first signs

The first signs an individual learns are special because they form the basis of an understanding of how signs may be used. They are also the most difficult signs to teach: learning later signs generally takes less time. The choice of the first sign is therefore especially important. Making a 'correct' choice may facilitate the teaching process. This chapter covers the first 10–20 signs. Its aim is *not* to provide a recommended list of signs, but rather to discuss the principles that should be applied when choosing signs.

Signs should be chosen on the basis of their general usefulness. The most important criteria to be taken into account are the needs, interests and desires of the individual who is to use them. It is therefore a good rule to make sure that the first signs are signs that the teacher knows – or has good reason to believe – the individual will wish to use. This will ensure motivation and attentiveness, and make it easier to understand the purpose of signing. The significance of these advantages cannot be valued too highly. Motivation, attentiveness and an understanding of the usefulness of communication are conditions that are often lacking in the education of individuals with extensive language and communication disorders.

There is general agreement that signs should be selected on the basis of their usefulness, but less agreement as to what is useful. Usefulness for the individuals' environment may often be placed before that of usefulness for the individuals. Usefulness implies that individuals are able to make themselves understood in such a way that they can initiate participation in activities. This type of usefulness is especially important for individuals who belong to the alternative language group, but is also the basis for choosing signs for individuals who belong to the other two groups.

For individuals who belong to the supportive language group, there may be specific objects or activities that are

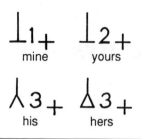

mine   yours

his   hers

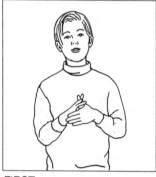

FIRST

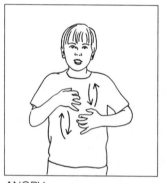

ANGRY

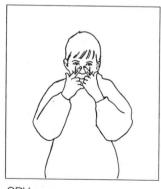

CRY

difficult to ask for or situations where they find it difficult to make themselves understood. If arguments over toys frequently occur, MINE, YOURS and HIS/HERS may be useful. FIRST may be used in the sense 'I had it first'. There are also examples where signs for emotions such as ANGRY and CRY ('sad') have proved useful among children with a difficult temper. However, it must be stressed that such words can be very difficult to teach, and if they are to be used as first signs, they should be taught to children with a good understanding of language.

Many individuals who belong to the expressive language group have a fairly good understanding of language. The purpose of the first signs is therefore not to teach them how the signs are used, but to instill them with a sense that the signs are useful. Communication boards are often not used in spontaneous communication (Glennen and Calculator, 1985; Harris, 1982), and many of the signs typically placed on the communication board may not encourage their use (Figure 30). The first signs should therefore give individuals better access to the activities and objects that they want.

Other people also need to learn one or more specific signs. Family members and others in close contact with individuals need to be able to make themselves understood, and the usefulness of signs should also be seen in terms of these needs. For the purposes of upbringing, parents and those in close contact with children need to be able to explain what the children are allowed to do, what is dangerous and how best to behave. They also need to be able to communicate what is going to happen, since the behavioural problems and anxiety experienced by linguistically impaired people are often related to their lack of understanding of what other people want them to do (Frith, 1989). This means that individuals should be taught to understand signal and command signs, which may make life easier and eliminate misunderstandings and conflicts.

Existing communication

Only seldom will individuals totally lack communication skills when the communication teaching begins. Existing communication skills should be taken into account when selecting signs. This communication has generally developed through interaction between individuals and their family, and it may have taken many years to establish sounds, gestures and facial expressions, etc. that the family and others who know them well are able to understand. It is also essential that this 'private' communication is used as a starting point, so that the individual begins by learning new ways to express things he is already capable of communicating.

Figure 30. *Examples of communication boards that do not encourage use. (Feallock, 1958; McDonald and Schultz, 1973).*

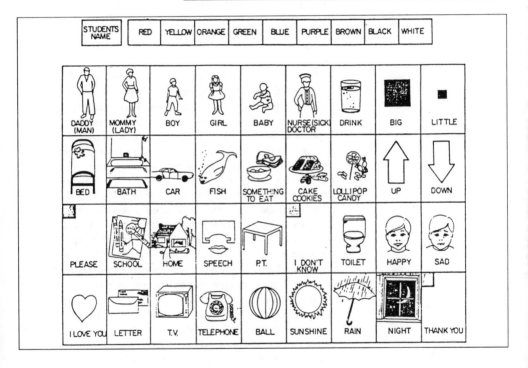

For example, if a boy smacks his lips in order to express the fact that he would like some raisins, the sign RAISIN should not be one of the first signs he learns. If the teacher had chosen to teach the boy the sign RAISIN, this would mean he would have to unlearn what he already knew, that is, he would be robbed of some of the communication skills he already possessed. The aim of the teaching is to provide more communication skills, not to change the form of those that already exist. Part of the preliminary teaching will therefore consist of training the professionals to understand the communicative expressions the individual already possesses. It is only at a later stage, when the sign vocabulary has been expanded, that the original communication

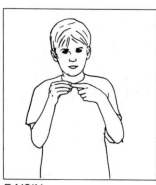

RAISIN

raisins

can be replaced with other, more commonly used signs. Individuals who receive communication aids will generally continue to use vocalisation, gestures, their gaze etc., even though graphic signs or script form their conventional communication.

Choosing between expressive and comprehension signs

The objective of augmentative communication teaching is to provide individuals with a better means of expressing themselves and understanding what other people are communicating. In expressive training individuals are taught to express himself to others. In comprehension training they are taught to understand what other people are communicating to them.

In reality, most language and communication teaching consists of both comprehension training and expressive training. However, there are both theoretical and practical arguments for giving priority to either comprehension or expressive use in the first stages of teaching. Among other things, the theoretical arguments stem from different views on the relationship between language and cognition in human development. Those who give priority to comprehension training base their arguments on the theory that children must first acquire concepts before they can learn words or signs. From this point of view, it is natural to begin with concept training and assume that the signs will be used once the concepts have been understood. It has generally been assumed that comprehension always precedes use in language development, but nowadays it has become more common to hold that expressive use and comprehension developed simultaneously and complement one another. Sometimes individuals' use of a sign or word will be more advanced than their comprehension of that same sign or word, at other times comprehension is acquired first (Clark, 1982). A developmental order of concepts and words may vary, and children can learn concepts by using words or signs.

In instances where it is necessary to give priority to one or other form of teaching, it is, in our opinion, most productive to give emphasis to expressive training. There are several reasons for this. There is no clear relationship between individuals' understanding of how other people use a sign and their beginning to use that sign for themselves in the same way. On the other hand, use of a sign implies teaching in what the sign means. When others react to the sign an individual uses, their reactions will over time make it possible for him or her to understand how the sign is used. It is therefore more likely that expressive training will lead to comprehension than that comprehension training will lead to expressive use.

In traditional teaching of children with delayed language development, comprehension training does not lead to use (Leonard, 1981). Autistic children who had been taught expressive use both understood and used manual signs better than autistic children who had been taught comprehension (Watters, Wheeler and Watters, 1981).

In a study of children with Down's syndrome, Romski and Ruder (1984) found that teaching using manual signs and speech did not produce better results than teaching where only speech was used. This finding is unusual because the use of supportive signs among this group has generally produced very good results (see for instance Johansson, 1987; Kotkin, Simpson and Desanto, 1978; Prevost, 1983; Rostad, 1989). What distinguishes this study from others in terms of method is that *the children themselves did not use signs*. It was the teacher who used signs and speech, or speech alone. This study reinforces the assumption that motor performance plays a role in the acquisition of manual signs, and it emphasises how important it is that individuals performs the signs themselves.

Another significant reason for giving priority to expressive training instead of comprehension training is that expressive training directly teaches individuals to influence their surroundings. In comprehension training the teacher takes the initiative, while the linguistically impaired individual provides the teacher with answers or carries out instructions. Expressive training shifts the communicative initiative to the individual. A lack of communicative initiative is one of the most fundamental problems among individuals with extensive language disorders. By teaching these individuals expressive use, there is greater reason to hope that communicative initiative on their part will be encouraged.

The fact that expressive training is given priority does not mean that comprehension training has no place in the teaching. Especially once a good many signs have been learned, it may be productive to teach expressive use and comprehension of the same signs simultaneously.

For some groups of disabled people, comprehension training should be given priority. This is especially the case for girls with Rett's syndrome, whose most characteristic feature is apraxia, i.e. an inability to perform voluntary actions. Girls with Rett's syndrome are almost totally incapable of expressing themselves, and the primary aim of the teaching should therefore be to increase their understanding of language and everyday activities.

Neither does an emphasis on expressive training imply

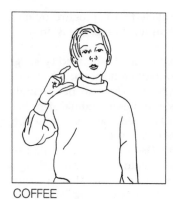

COFFEE

that comprehension is of no significance when choosing signs. It is quicker for individuals to learn to use signs that correspond to known words than it is to learn signs corresponding to unknown words (Clarke, Remington and Light, 1986). An understanding of the situation may also facilitate sign acquisition. There are examples showing that in the early stages of normal language development children use words in situations with which they are familiar. For example, Bloom's daughter only used *car* about the cars she saw from the window (Bloom, 1973). In terms of sign or speech teaching, it is similarly easiest to begin learning signs or words in known situations, where the function of the signs or words is known.

General and specific signs

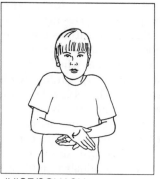

JUICE/SQUASH

In our opinion the first expressive signs should be *specific*, i.e. related to objects and actions. The alternative is to link the signs to *classes* of objects, activities or events. COFFEE, SQUASH, WEAVE and SEW may be regarded as specific signs while DRINK and WORK are *general*. For example, WORK may be used to indicate sewing, weaving or cutting grass.

The reason for choosing specific rather than general signs whenever this is practically feasible is to avoid problems that may arise when individuals learn new signs. If, for example, individuals have learned the sign DRINK in an situation where they are given squash each time they use the

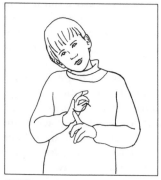

SEW

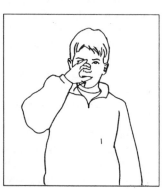

DRINK

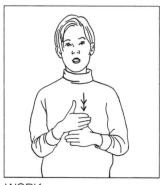

WORK

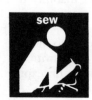

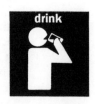

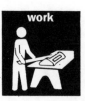

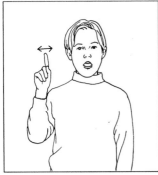

WHAT

sign, it may subsequently be difficult to teach them to use the sign SQUASH. In order to teach SQUASH, the teacher must either combine DRINK and SQUASH to form a sign sentence, or perhaps introduce a practice where the individuals begin by using DRINK, the teacher then asks WHAT and the individuals answer SQUASH. The teaching process becomes laborious, and provides plenty of opportunities for misunderstanding. Learning a specific sign may also involve the unlearning of the general sign. This may be the case if an individual interprets the general sign as more specific than the teacher had intended: i.e. in a way that either partially or totally corresponded to the use of the specific sign. For example, someone might take DRINK to mean 'squash'. The chances that individuals will misunderstand are great, because it may be easy for them to interpret a general sign as a specific sign when the sign is used to denote an interesting object or activity.

Signal signs can be both specific and general, but in contrast to expressive signs the first signal signs will often be the ones that signal a general situation, such as FOOD before a meal, SPORT before physical activity and MUSIC before music therapy and other musical activities.

The aim of expressive teaching in the use of graphic and manual signs is that individuals should be able to give expression to wants and thoughts, and influence their environment in a way that is socially acceptable. They have to learn the consequences the sign may have. Each sign

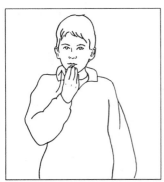

FOOD

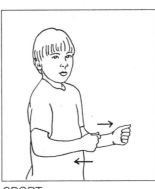

SPORT

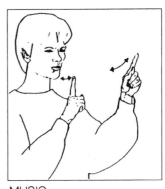

MUSIC

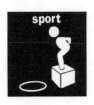

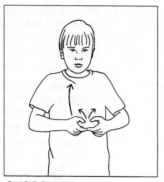

CHOCOLATE

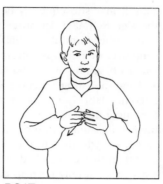

BOAT

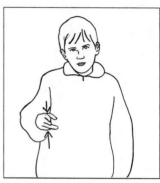

SCISSORS

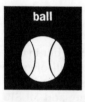

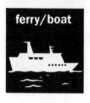

should have a different consequence, so that not all signs are interpreted as variations of one general sign. An individual who is given a piece of chocolate on performing the signs BALL, BOAT and SCISSORS when these objects are present will learn that BALL means 'chocolate' when there is a ball on the table, BOAT means 'chocolate' when there is a boat on the table, and SCISSORS means 'chocolate' when there is a pair of scissors on the table. Thus, the chocolate makes it difficult for the learner to understand the connection between BALL and the act of rolling or throwing a ball, between BOAT and playing with the boat in the bathtub, and between SCISSORS and the act of cutting paper.

A primary objective for individuals who belong to the expressive language group is that they should be able to initiate conversation and other forms of interaction. In addition, the signs they learn should cover a variety of situations and subjects. Useful general first signs are such signs as COME, LOOK, PLAY and TALK. With such general expressions, there is still a risk that individuals will remain passive and that the activities they take part in will chiefly be decided by others. In order to foster independence, they must be able to take the initiative in deciding activities, so specific signs such as BOOK, COMPUTER, DOLL and LORRY may also be useful early words for this group.

Repetitions

It is essential for all three groups that the signs chosen are ones that can be used fairly frequently. For the alternative language and supportive language group, it is important that the signs are repeated often enough for them to be learned. For example, the signs SWIM and RIDE are not particularly well suited to the early stages of expressive training because such activities occur only once a week, or even less. When the teaching takes place in the individual's natural environment, the best strategy is to use signs that

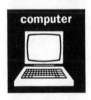

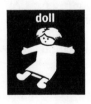

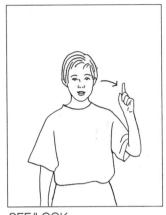
SEE/LOOK

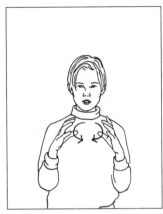
BALL

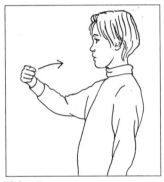
COME

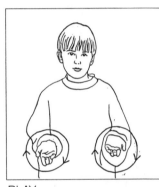
PLAY

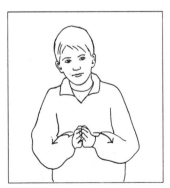
BOOK

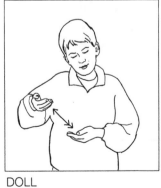
DOLL

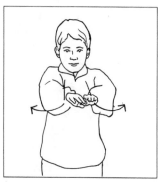

SWIM

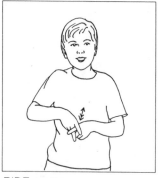

RIDE

can be used in connection with routine activities and other frequently repeated activities. Signs that are often used as first signs are the names of items of food, and other objects and activities that are not usually mentioned very often. In special training and planned teaching situations the teacher has greater control over how often the signs will be used, and it may be advantageous to design a situation that gives individuals the chance to learn such signs through named practice – on the condition that they do not become bored. Activities the individuals enjoy are easier to repeat in the natural environment.

Motor skills

The learner must be able to perform the sign so that it is easily understood. Manual signs place the greatest demands on motor skills, and they should not be used if motor disorders prevent their performance. Individuals should not have such great difficulty in performing the signs that their attention becomes focused on how the signs are articulated, losing track of their function.

Many people in need of augmentative communication are clumsy, and it may be difficult to recognise the manual signs they are performing. If an individual performs signs childishly or clumsily, the conversational partner may, for example, confuse such signs as FOOD and DRINK. A problem one often encounters is that the individual is unable to make the distinction in hand shape, with the result that both FOOD and DRINK are performed by leading the hand to the mouth without forming the hands into the specific shape required. It is therefore more practical to use THIRSTY instead of DRINK, since THIRSTY is performed with the hands in a different position relative to the individual's body. In this way, both signs may be used without placing too much emphasis on their articulation. It is the function, not the articulation, of the signs that should be emphasised; especially when teaching the first signs. CAR and MILK are two other signs that are frequently used but are difficult to distinguish from one another. DRIVE may be a better sign to use than CAR, because its articulation is easier to distinguish from that of MILK.

On occasions when it is not possible to find manual signs that are easy to perform, another strategy is to simplify the signs. However, it is important to be aware that simplifying the way the signs are articulated does not *always* make them easier to learn. Many individuals with extensive communication disorders find it easier to learn manual signs than graphic signs, even though graphic signs are always easier to perform. It seems that though the actual

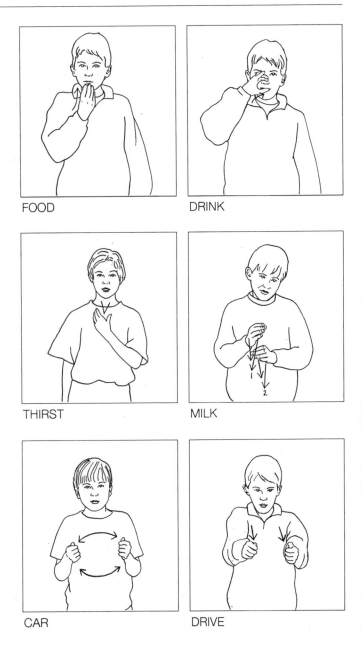

FOOD

DRINK

THIRST

MILK

CAR

DRIVE

motor production of manual signs – which differs for each sign – is an aid to distinguishing one sign from another. This also requires the signs to be different in terms of motor articulation.

There are no fixed rules about what distinguishes manual signs that are easy to learn from those that are difficult, but there are studies that give some clues about the type of simplification that should be made. The hand shapes should be simple, and the fingers should not have to be placed in unusual positions. Two-handed signs are easier to learn than one-handed signs. Symmetrical signs, i.e. signs where both hands perform the same movement, are easier to learn than asymmetrical signs, where the hands have different functions. It appears that touch is a good aid to learning and performing signs. Manual signs where the hands touch the body are easier to learn than signs where the hands are not in contact with the body. As might be expected, complex signs are more difficult to learn than signs with only one movement (Dennis et al., 1982). More information is needed before it is known how signs should best be simplified, and individual differences should be taken into consideration. It makes good sense to take these circumstances into account, however, both when selecting and simplifying manual signs.

The primary motor skill required when using graphic signs is the ability to point. Accuracy of movement determines the size of signs required, and thus how many signs there will be room for on the communication board. The location on the communication board is important. It may be necessary to use only some areas of the board (Figure 31). When individuals begin sign training, it is essential that they have as few problems pointing as possible, so that they will experience positive results immediately. People in the individuals' environment will not be accustomed to using signs either. The fact that individuals are able to point reasonably quickly may help conversational partners to break former communication patterns in which they wholly dominated the communicative situation.

Figure 31. *Boards may have an unusual design owing to perceptual or motor limitations on the part of the user.*

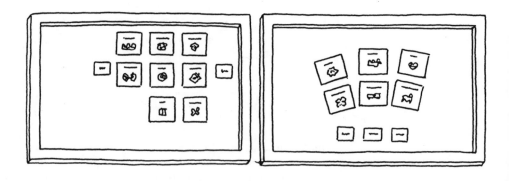

Perception

The ability to perceive sensory impressions is of crucial importance, for the choice of both sign system and individual signs. A visually impaired individual may have difficulty in distinguishing between and perceiving manual signs used by others. Sight is also an aid when learning expressive signs. Manual signs the individual is able to see while performing them may be easier to learn than others (Luftig, 1984). Visual acuity will determine the size of graphic signs, and the choice of them. Reduced visual acuity may make it difficult for the individual to distinguish between graphic signs that resemble one another. In cases where individuals have lost part of their field of vision or are blind in one eye, it may be necessary to use only part of the communication board. With individuals who have severe visual impairments, communication aids that utilise artificial speech may be used. Such communication aids may utilise several switches or a concept keyboard where each square has a different texture (Mathy-Laikko et al., 1989).

In order to make graphic systems accessible for people with visual impairments, sculptured three-dimensional PIC signs have been produced that enable individuals to perceive the signs by feeling them with their fingers. These may be of use to people with partially impaired vision, who use the sense of touch as a supplement to sight. For individuals who are totally dependent on perceiving the differences between signs by touch, though, PIC signs of this sort are not particularly suitable. Perceiving forms with one's fingers is difficult. Many of the differences that are easy to perceive using sight are not as easy to perceive with the aid of touch. Premack's word bricks are probably better in this respect because they consist of easily recognisable forms and can be manipulated for further investigation. However, it is better to use a distinctive graphic sign system, which takes into account the possibilities and limitations offered by visual impairment.

It is not only visual disorders in the usual sense that are of significance for the perception of visual impressions. Brain damage may make it difficult to process and interpret visual sensations. For example, *stimulus overselectivity* may make it difficult to distinguish between graphic signs. Stimulus overselectivity means that the individual uses only one or few of the available cues when identifying an object (Løvaas, Koegel and Schreibman, 1979). If one changes the attributes that the individual uses as cues for recognising a particular object, he or she will fail to recognise that object. Stimulus overselectivity is common among people with severe mental handicap. If it is suspected, one should

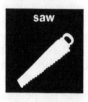

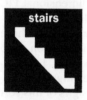

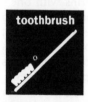

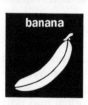

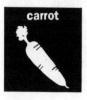

should choose graphic signs which, owing to their common features, are probably not as easy for the individual to mix up.

If the individual has problems seeing the differences between the PIC signs or between signs in other graphic sign systems, it may be necessary to simplify or change the form of the signs. This can be done with the aid of a black felt-tip pen.

If the individual has some understanding of speech, it is important to utilise this understanding. For example, people with developmental dysphasia often have difficulty distinguishing between words that sound alike (homonyms). Care should therefore be taken so that signs that correspond to similar sounding words are not chosen.

Iconicity

Iconicity is regarded as a condition that facilitates the acquisition of both manual and graphic signs.

> *Iconicity* means that there is a similarity between the performance or appearance of a sign and obvious features of the object or action the sign is used to describe. Iconicity is measured in terms of *transparency* and *translucency*.

> *Transparency* indicates the ease with which people who are unfamiliar with the sign are able to guess the meaning of the sign. Transparency is the feature one usually associates with iconicity.

> *Translucency* indicates the ease with which one can perceive a relationship between a sign's meaning and its performance.

A sign can be translucent even though the relationship perceived is not the true connection between the sign's sense and its form. For example, GIRL in American sign language is highly translucent because many people perceive a connection between the way the sign is performed – the thumb is stroked across the cheek – and the fact that girls have soft cheeks. The sign actually originates from the fact that girls in the United States in the last century wore bonnets that were held in place by a band attached under their chin. The stroking movement comes from the bonnet band (Klima and Bellugi, 1979).

Manual signs

The relationship between iconicity and the acquisition of manual signs depends on the diagnostic group being studied, and whether transparency or translucency is used as a measure of iconicity (Doherty, 1985).

There is no clear connection between how easy it is for

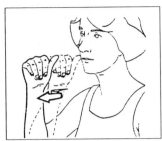

GIRL (American Sign Language)

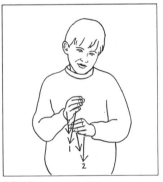

MILK

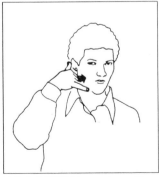

TELEPHONE (American Sign Language)

it is to learn them. The transparency of manual signs, measured by the adults guessing at the signs' gloss, is not always significant in terms of the ease with which those signs may be acquired. Deaf children do not learn more iconic manual signs in their early development than one would expect on the basis of the share of iconic signs found in American Sign Language (Bonvillian, Orlansky and Novack. 1981). Brown (1977) found that children learned to recognise transparent manual signs more quickly than non-transparent ones, while others have had less success in finding a link between transparency and recognition (Miller, 1987) or production (Trasher and Bray, 1984) of manual signs among mentally handicapped individuals. Goosens' (1983) found, however, that there was a connection between transparency and recognition of manual signs if mentally handicapped individuals were also used to establish whether or not the signs were transparent. The fact that transparency plays a role in the recognition of learned but forgotten signs is not surprising, since the ability to guess the meanings of signs follows from the definition of transparency. Since one may guess signs one has forgotten, the transparency will always lead to a higher score than instances where it was not as easy to remember the names one had forgotten. But signs that are transparent for some people – for example, university students – are not necessarily so for others – such as linguistically impaired nursery school children. MILK was perhaps fairly transparent for children during the last century because many of them had seen a cow being milked by hand. Today there are few children who would associate the sign with milking.

The differences that exist in the perception of translucency manifest themselves clearly in a study of 100 American manual signs for object words that are often used in the teaching of mentally handicapped individuals. A group of normally developed 6-year-olds rated only one sign (TELEPHONE) as being highly translucent. Hearing and deaf students rated 26 signs as being highly translucent. For the children and the hearing students 55 and 48 signs, respectively, were given a low translucency rating, while the deaf students rated only 16 signs as being of low translucency (Griffith and Robinson, 1981).

With regard to the use of manual signs, research has not found that a high or low degree of translucency plays a role in the ease with which severely handicapped individuals learn signs (Kohl, 1981). In terms of recognition of manual signs, it has been found that signs that were rated as being highly translucent are remembered better than those that were rated as having a low degree of translucency (Griffith and Robinson, 1981). This is to be expected, since many highly translucent signs will also be highly transparent.

It is not surprising that university students benefit from translucency when remembering signs. Perceiving a relationship makes it easier for them to recall a particular sign, and the establishment of such connections is a memory technique that is commonly used (cf. Klima and Bellugi, 1979; Luria, 1969). For normally developed 3-year-olds, however, it seems that iconicity is of no help when recognising manual signs (Miller, 1987). On occasions when mentally handicapped people do not learn translucent manual signs any quicker than non-translucent signs, this may be due to the fact that they lack the skills needed for them to be able to utilise such similarities, i.e. they are unable to see the connection between the sign they are making and a specific aspect of the object or action represented in the performance of the sign.

There is thus little to support the theory that iconicity facilitates the acquisition of the first manual signs by small children and mentally handicapped people. However, iconicity does facilitate recognition and production among other adults. Choosing iconic manual signs may therefore help create a more responsive language environment by increasing the chances that the sign will be recognised, and will help the adult to remember what the sign is supposed to express. For this reason, iconic signs should be chosen where there is a choice of signs that otherwise seem equally functional and easy to learn.

Graphic signs

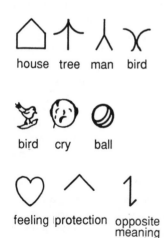

house tree man bird

bird cry ball

feeling protection opposite meaning

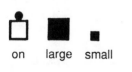

on large small

When assessing iconicity in graphic sign systems, pictorial similarity is clearer. Many of the sign systems consist of more or less stylised drawings, and even drawings that are not part of a graphic sign system have been called iconic (cf. Hurlbut et al., 1982). Signs of this type are said to be *pictographic*. A number of graphic signs are not pictographic in the strictest sense of the word, but portray an object or action that is usually associated with what the sign is used to describe. Such signs are often said to be *ideographic*. There are also graphic systems with little or no iconicity, such as Premack's word bricks and Lexigrams.

Roughly speaking, the Blissymbols and Rebus signs that are described as pictographic are transparent, while the signs that are characterised as ideographic are translucent. The Blissymbols HOUSE, TREE, MAN and BIRD are regarded as pictographic; so too are the Rebus signs BIRD, CRY and BALL. The Blissymbols FEELING, PROTECTION and OPPOSITE are ideographic, though, as are the Rebus signs ON, LARGE and SMALL. HELP is a typically ideographic PCS sign.

All PIC signs should be pictographic, but signs such as

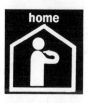

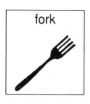

HELP, HOME and FRIENDS are nonetheless classified as ideographic. This is a natural result of the fact that not all words are easy to illustrate. Although this has not been studied, there is reason to believe that iconic graphic signs that correspond to object words (nouns) are transparent, while iconic graphic signs that correspond to verbs and other classes of words are more translucent. In all probability there are also relatively more iconic signs among object groups than other word classes (Figure 32).

There are no comparisons of graphic signs within a single system. Attempts to ascertain the significance of iconicity have been concentrated on comparing the various systems. The results from such studies show for the most part that systems with a greater proportion of iconic signs are easier to learn than systems with many non-iconic signs. Blissymbols are generally easier to learn than Premack's word bricks, and Rebus signs are easier to learn than Blissymbols. The differences reported are chiefly concerned with associative learning and recognition of the signs, i.e. that the subjects being investigated have to remember which signs correspond to particular words. Hurlbut and his colleagues (1982) found, however, that mentally handicapped individuals also used drawings more spontaneously than Blissymbols.

Based on comparisons of systems, it appears that iconic graphic signs should be chosen as a starting point. However, it should be said that arriving at such a conclusion is not a simple matter. Severely mentally handicapped individuals are not always able to perceive what a picture is supposed to represent. This may mean that figurative differences which seem great to most people because they convey meaning are not so clear for individuals who are unable to perceive the content of the picture. For example, some individuals may see little difference between the PCS signs FORK and TOOTHBRUSH if they are unaware of the objects' function and do not notice the prongs on the fork and the bristles on the toothbrush. There is reason to believe that many severely mentally handicapped individuals have difficulty in perceiving this type of difference, perhaps because of stimulus overselectivity or poor visual scanning strategies (cf. Lyon and Ross, 1984).

Recognising objects in pictures is only a small step in the development of pictorial perception. Perceiving action in pictures is learned at a later stage than the perception of objects (Kose et al., 1983), and in view of the fact that many mentally handicapped individuals have difficulty in recognising objects in pictures (Dixon, 1981), one should be even more cautious about taking their perception of other sorts of picture content for granted. It is not easy to express an action, preposition, etc. pictorially and unambiguously.

Figure 32. *Graphic signs that correspond to different word groups.*

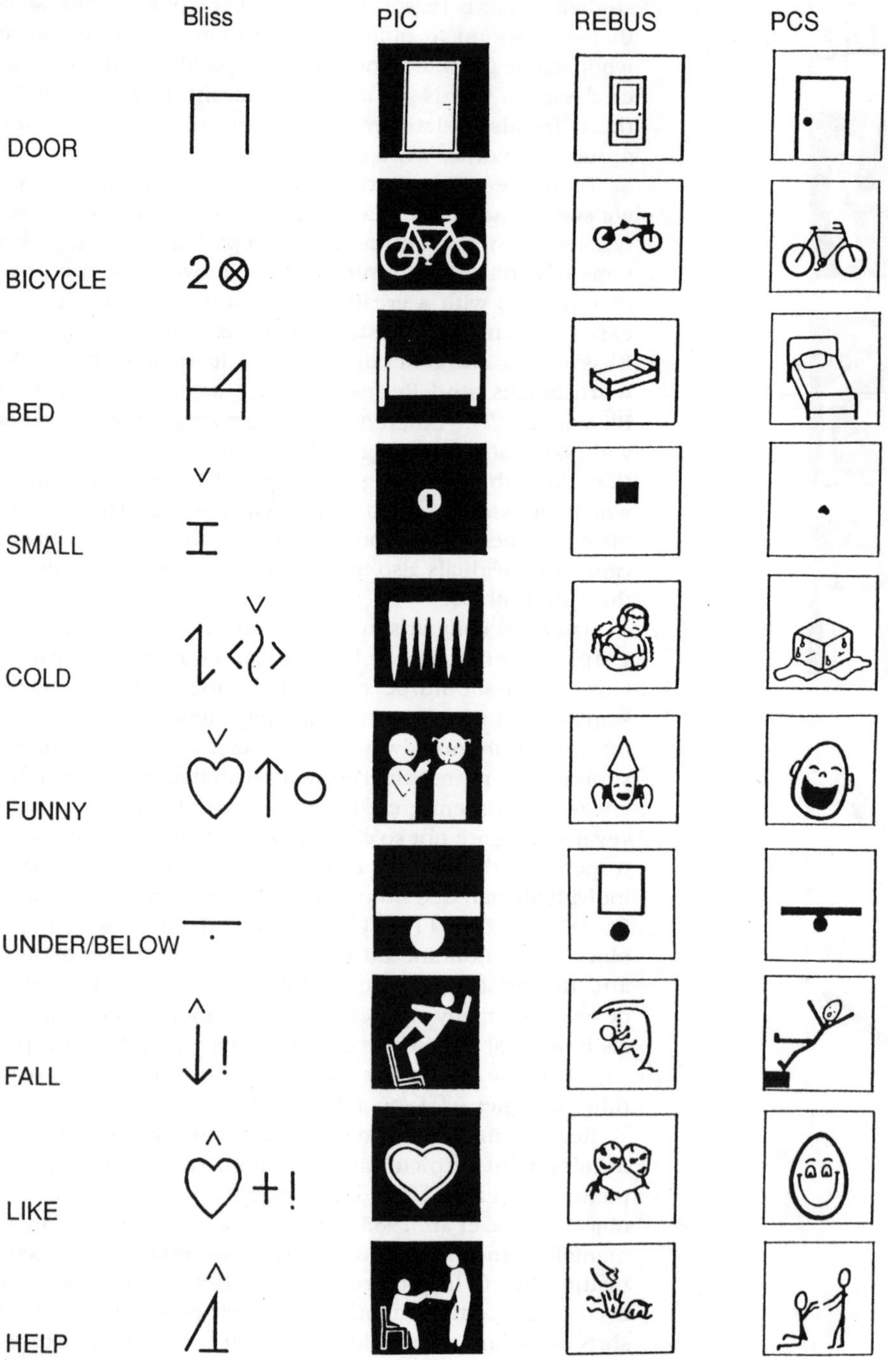

	Bliss	PIC	REBUS	PCS
DOOR				
BICYCLE	2⊗			
BED				
SMALL				
COLD				
FUNNY				
UNDER/BELOW				
FALL				
LIKE				
HELP				

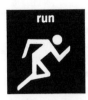

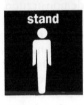

If the sign learners do not understand that a sign is the name of an action, or is supposed to signal one, they may perhaps perceive it as depicting an object. The PIC signs RUN, JUMP and STAND may just as easily be perceived as 'man' or 'human'. Pictorial accuracy may only make the signs appear more similar, which is more likely to confuse learners than to help them.

This discussion is not intended to be an argument against the use of iconic graphic signs in early teaching. There is reason to believe that such signs will facilitate the learning process for individuals who have developed the necessary pictorial comprehension. However, for many mentally handicapped individuals this is not the case. If individuals appear unable to perceive the figurative pictorial content that has been stressed in the choice of signs, then the signs are not iconic for them and iconicity therefore cannot make the learning process easier. It becomes more important to ensure that individual can distinguish between the forms found in the signs that will be used, which may be done by traditional teaching of discrimination. If individuals are able to distinguish between iconic graphic signs, it is advantageous to use them, since this helps to ensure that other people in the environment will react to their comprehension and expressive use.

The wish to illustrate and make clear the significance of the signs can sometimes produce very unfortunate results. For example, YES and NO are usually illustrated with a smiling face and a sad face. This does not correspond at all well to the use of these two words. These faces are clearly misleading when used in reply to such questions as *Are you sad? Are you angry? Did he go? Is it raining?* or *Is it broken?* The end result may be that individuals will generally regard the NO sign as negative and the YES sign as positive. There is also reason to believe that the conversational partners of children will take notice of the drawings themselves and use them to express whether the child is happy or sad.

Simple and complex concepts

When one begins to teach language to individuals with extensive communication disorders, it is necessary to take into account what the learners can understand of the signs. However, in such circumstances it is not always clear which concepts are difficult and which are easy. For example, 'mummy' and 'daddy' can hardly be regarded as particularly difficult concepts, but it may nonetheless be difficult to teach comprehension and expressive use of the signs MUMMY and DADDY.

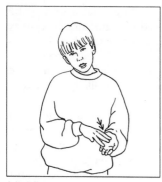

MUMMY

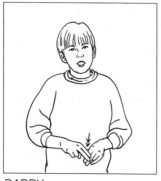

DADDY

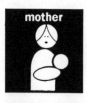

Instead of speaking in terms of simple and difficult concepts, it may be better to speak of circumstances that make such concepts either difficult or easy to teach. Lahey and Bloom (1977) place great emphasis on 'ease of demonstration' when choosing first signs, and cite, for example, the difficulties of demonstrating an individual's inner state as an argument for excluding signs that express feelings when choosing a first vocabulary for linguistically impaired children.

When Lahey and Bloom prepared their guidelines they probably had in mind children with delayed language development and less extensive disorders. They appear to assume that a child with a communication disorder can learn by observing other people, and ease of demonstration may thus be interpreted in a fairly literal sense. This is the case for many individuals who belong to the expressive language group, but for people with more extensive language disorders, the 'ease of demonstration' of the first sign is a question of designing a situation where the relationship between the sign and changes in the situation is as clear as possible. When teaching signal signs this means that the situation in which the sign is taught must be clear and defined. When teaching expressive signs the objects and activities should be reasonably similar in function or design over time, so that they are recognisable each time they are used.

It is also essential that the first signs are not too similar in terms of content, so that they do not cause confusion. However, determining whether signs are similar in terms of content is no easy task. Similarity may imply that both signs belong to the same category or that one is a sub-set of the other. For example, MILK and JUICE are both a form of DRINK. APPLE and BANANA are FRUIT, while POTATO and SAUSAGE are DINNER. All of these are FOOD. It is common for two or three things from the same category to be used in a given situation, but one should try to avoid a situation where one sign is part of another. FOOD and DRINK are often used as signal signs while other words for food are being practised, but these two signs are not used in such a way that the other food signs function as sub-categories of them. The meaning of FOOD might just as well be described as 'eat' or 'You may have something to eat now'. Similarly, DRINK is used to signal 'You may have something to drink now'. In this way these signs denote *domains* where different signs may be used.

When the first sign teaching is initiated, the individuals will not learn a general use of the words such as that found among competent language users. For them a word such as *sausage* will be used in a variety of combinations; *smoked sausage, sausage roll, liver sausage*, etc. Individuals with

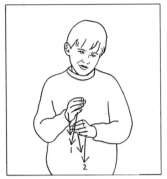

MILK

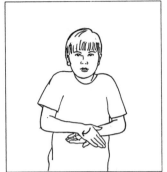

JUICE/SQUASH

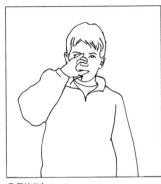

DRINK

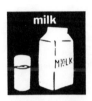

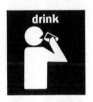

communication disorders will first learn a *limited use* of the signs. SAUSAGE, for example, will best be translated with the phrase 'I want a hot dog'. Using SAUSAGE to say 'There is a sausage' or SAUSAGE RED to say 'I want a red sausage' or 'the sausage is Danish' is a skill that will be learned at a later stage. This depends on whether the sign SAUSAGE has been used in situations that are functionally different. If an individual mixes up the signs TROUSERS and SHIRT after practising these signs in a single situation (Doherty, 1985), there is reason to believe that he or she has not systematically identified each of these garments with the particular routine of putting on either trousers or a shirt. The situation in which the dressing has taken place has not contained sufficient cues for the individual to be able to distinguish between them.

Another way of finding words with a conceptual content that individuals ought to find easy to learn has been to register the words used by children learning to speak. It has been assumed that these words must correspond to concepts that people with poor communicative skills have or are in the process of learning, and that they are therefore be the most suitable ones to teach as first words, both for normal small children in the early stages of development and for individuals with extensive communication disorders who acquire language at a later stage. On the basis of their assumptions about what is expressed in early language development, Lahey and Bloom (1977) list six rules for choosing first words.

Object words (objects, people and places) can be chosen relatively freely, based on the situations the individual experiences.

Relational words (verbs, adjectives, prepositions, etc.) should be chosen so that they can be used with all or a large number of objects.

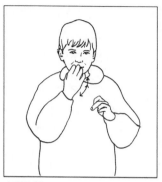

APPLE

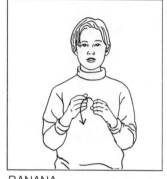

BANANA

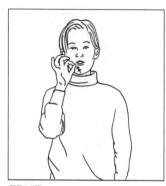

FRUIT

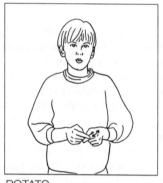

POTATO

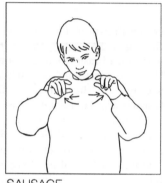

SAUSAGE

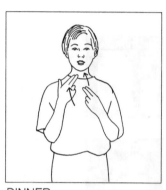

DINNER

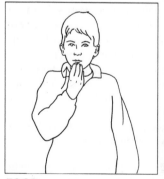

FOOD

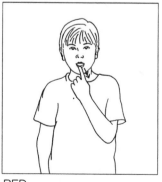

RED

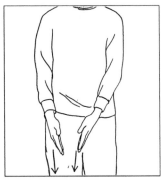

TROUSERS

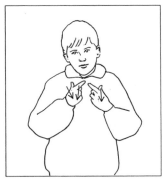

SHIRT

Avoid *words for inner feelings* as these are difficult to demonstrate, and thus to teach.

Avoid *Yes* and *No* as expressions of affirmation and denial. *No* can be used to express other important conditions.

Avoid pronouns, which are usually acquired at a later stage. Use *mummy* and *daddy* and people's names instead.

Avoid colours and opposites (*big – small*). Use only one element of such pairs since opposites are acquired at a late stage and may confuse the child. It is better to use the word *not* instead, for example, *not-big* instead of *small*.

Most of these points make good sense. One should not, however, link the difference between object words and relational words with word classes. A word class may only be defined on the basis of the function that the words belonging to that class have in the sentence, and as long as an individual is not combining words to make sentences, there is little sense in saying that a sign belongs to a specific word class. Thus, JUMP and WALK may not be regarded as belonging to a different word class from ICE CREAM and GRAPE unless they are used to express different functions in multiple sign utterances.

Emphasising NO to express rejection or refusal, non-existence, cessation of an activity and a ban on a particular activity, seems to be academically motivated. In the early stages of sign teaching NO should be avoided as an expression of non-existence since adults should be able to use NO in order to deny the individual an activity or thing, without the child misunderstanding. For example, if a girl says CHOCOLATE and the teacher says NO, she may interpret this as meaning that there is no chocolate. If there is a bar of chocolate lying on the table, or the girl has seen the teacher put one in the cupboard, this may lead her to believe that she has not been understood and she will therefore continue to say CHOCOLATE. Because she is used to being misunderstood, this is a reasonable assumption on her part. It is useful to be able to express the non-existence of an object, especially if the individual notices that a particular object is missing. However, GONE is a better choice of word than NO. It is questionable, though, whether GONE will be used any differently from the words GET, GIVE or HELP. These signs may also be used to obtain something that does not exist in a particular situation. It is a matter of finding out which sign is easiest to teach, and GONE may well prove to be the most appropriate one.

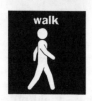

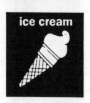

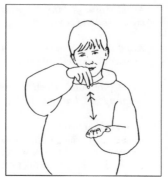

JUMP

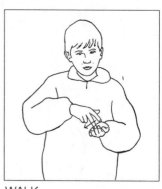

WALK

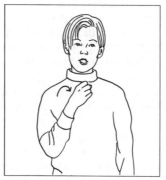

ICE CREAM

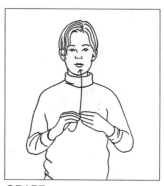

GRAPE

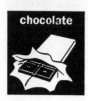

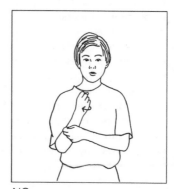

NO

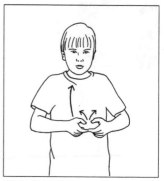

CHOCOLATE

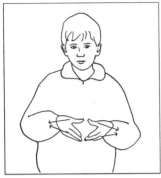

GONE

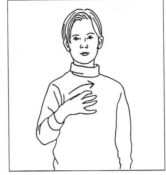

GET

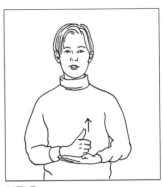

HELP

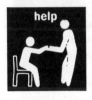

What to expect

The teacher's expectations of the first stage of sign teaching will differ depending on which of the three groups is being taught, and on the stated aims of the teaching. Many individuals who belong to the expressive language group have a good enough understanding of language at the start of the teaching that there is good reason to expect them to learn quickly. However, it may take a long time before the signs are used spontaneously, which is the aim of the continued teaching. The supportive language group will also be expected to make rapid progress, since many in the group will be able to use a number of words and have a certain degree of language comprehension. The people with the greatest difficulties are found in the alternative language group, and it is here one finds the greatest degree of uncertainty in terms of teaching progression. Even though it seems that most individuals acquire some communicative skills when they are taught to use graphic or manual signs, there are great variations. Wills (1981) summarises 17 studies of 118 people. Nine individuals learned no signs, while the greatest number of signs acquired was 24 for each month of teaching. The average was three new signs for each month of teaching.

Even though the teaching is functional and takes place in the individual's natural environment, it may sometimes take several months before the signs are used spontaneously. Older people with communication disorders in particular will have a long history of learned dependence, helplessness and passivity. For individuals with extensive disorders, it is important to continue the training for long enough to allow the individual time in which to learn. When the teaching goes well and the individual begins to speak, it is important that the teaching does not stop. There are countless examples showing that signs help autistic and mentally handicapped children to find the word they wish to say, and stopping sign teaching at too early a stage may make the communication worse.

Chapter 9
Further development

Once an individual is able to use the first 10–20 signs consistently both spontaneously and in the teaching situation, the character of the teaching will change. For many individuals belonging to the alternative language group, the preliminary teaching will function as a test period because the course of development will be impossible to predict with any degree of certainty. Once the first signs have been learned, the teaching may become more flexible. An increased repertoire provides greater freedom of choice between the various teaching methods and enables greater versatility. This will also place new demands on the teacher. It is particularly important to have long-term aims and teaching strategies that prompt the learning of new language skills.

The objectives of this continued development are the same for all three groups: to teach new signs, lay the basis for the combination of signs to produce sentences and foster participation in conversations (see Chapter 10). However, these three aims will receive varying degrees of emphasis, depending on which group is being taught. The major difference will be between the expressive language group and the other two groups.

The alternative and supportive language groups

Building a vocabulary

When choosing new signs, emphasis is generally placed on individuals being able to communicate in as many situations as possible. They should be taught to use signs in new situations, so that it is possible for them to use signs throughout the day. This type of approach may be called

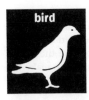

surface-oriented. Another approach is to teach individuals new signs related to situations that are already used in the sign teaching. The individuals will learn to use more than one sign from within the same topic or domain. This approach may be called *domain-oriented*. A domain-oriented expansion of sign vocabulary provides the basis for a more profound learning than that provided by surface-oriented expansion. A domain-oriented teaching programme may also enhance conversational skills because it gives individuals the opportunity to say more about the same subject.

> Jack is a 36-year-old mentally handicapped man. He is interested in birds, especially those in the park, so the domain BIRD is expanded with DUCK, WING, BEAK and FLY.

One of the best ways to increase the sign vocabulary is to combine the teaching of new signs with the teaching of new skills and activities. New comprehension signs can be taught by using new signs together with new activities, and by using signs as markers to signal new activities.

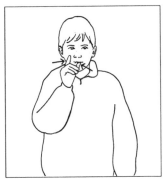

BIRD

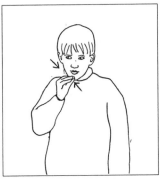

DUCK

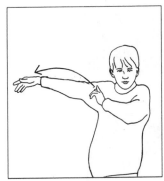

WING

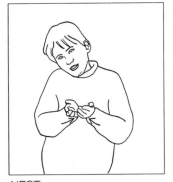

NEST

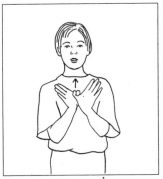

FLY

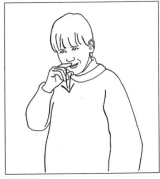

BEAK

ring/quoit

glass

spoon

fork

knife

Paul is a 5-year-old boy with a developmental language impairment. He enjoys throwing a ball, playing snap and taking part in other games. He is keen on playing a variation on the game of quoits but annoys the other children by trying to take the hoops when it is their turn. When it is his turn he is guided to make the sign RING before he is given the quoits.

The comprehension signs are naturally a mixture of signal signs and instructions. Some of the instructions are command signs, but *requests for action* gradually become more commonplace since the main aim of giving instructions is no longer to control problematic behaviour. Also, naming and commenting on objects and activities gradually becomes more commonplace.

Learning signs in fixed routines both facilitates the introduction of these routines and makes it easier for individuals to understand the signs, since they know which activity is going to follow.

Carol is a 20-year-old mentally handicapped girl. She usually helps lay the table and this activity is signalled with the sign LAY-TABLE. Plates, glasses and cutlery are placed on the table. Carol places these on the table one piece at a time and always in the same order; plates, glasses, forks, knives and spoons. She is guided to

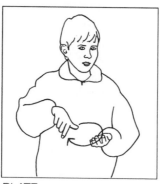

PLATE

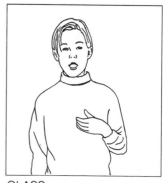

GLASS

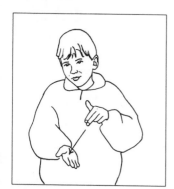

FORK

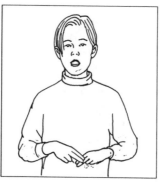

KNIFE

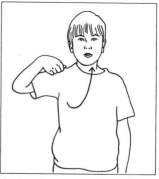

SPOON

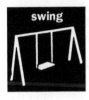

perform each of the signs every time she is given one of the objects.

It is also possible to use signal signs while carrying out an activity with the learner. If the activities are familiar ones and are repeated frequently, they provide good situations for sign teaching.

Among other strategies, the strategy of reacting to marker-controlled anticipatory behaviour is suitable as a means of increasing the number of expressive signs. The teacher can use a signal sign as a domain sign to give an individual the choice of at least two activities. The choice is made by training expressive signs. This form of domain-oriented teaching is available not only in situations where the individual wants something or wishes to do something but also in connection with naming.

> Irene is a 15-year-old autistic girl. She is fond of crafts and is being taught embroidery and knitting. Her craft lessons are signalled by the sign WORK. When her teacher brings out a basket of materials she is given the choice between SEW and KNIT.

One important aspect of domain-oriented teaching is that since several signs are linked to the same general situation, it encourages the individual to delineate the use of the signs. This helps to increase the length of social interaction within a framework that is familiar for the individual.

In both expressive training and comprehension training, an appropriate way of beginning the process of sign expansion is to utilise signs that can be used to represent several activities that have one or more features in common. For example, OUT may be used to designate all sorts of outdoor activities. However, it is important that this sign does not interfere with the learning of other specific signs for outdoor activities that the individuals enjoy. SWING and SLIDE are examples of specific outdoor activities. Therefore, OUT should first be learned in situations where these other specific signs are not used. The best way to do this is to create a situation where OUT requires the individuals to choose between two outdoor activities, so that OUT will not be confused with signs that are used to represent a specific activity. This implies that the teacher should begin by teaching the individuals to choose between two outdoor activities and then use OUT as a domain sign. Once OUT has been established, its use can be expanded to include more activities.

Contrasts between signs

When children learn to speak normally, it appears that they automatically assume that different words also have differ-

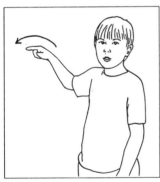

OUT

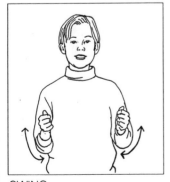

SWING

ent uses (Clark, 1983). However, one should not immediately infer that individuals with severe communication disorders will likewise automatically assume that the signs they are being taught are used differently. This supposition has nonetheless given rise to a strategy of exclusion as a means of introducing new signs when teaching comprehension to people with severe mental handicap. The teaching consists of giving the individuals a particular type of food when a manual sign is presented. Once they have learned to respond to the sign by taking the food, they are shown a new type of food together with the one they have already learned. The sign for the new type of food is then presented. The individuals respond to the new sign by taking the new food type, because they exclude the food type for which they already know the sign. For example, MEAT is introduced together with DRINK, with which they are familiar, CRISPS/POTATO CHIPS together with CAKE and TOAST together with EGG (McIlvane et al., 1984). This method would seem best suited to comprehension training, but with some changes it could be used for expressive training. Exclusion is also conceivable as a strategy for teaching the sign HELP by presenting new, attractive objects together

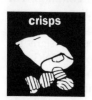

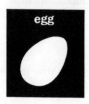

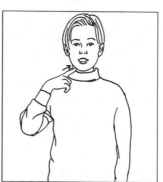

MEAT

DRINK

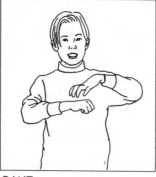

CAKE

EGG

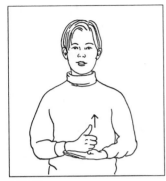

HELP

with objects with which the individuals are already familiar (in order to make it easier for them to understand that signs should be used).

If the tendency to perceive contrasts between signs is a robust phenomenon, this will be of great practical and theoretical significance. It implies, for example, that when individuals appear unable to distinguish between the use of two signs, it is not due to the fact that they perceive them as being 'synonymous', i.e. as having the same meaning, but because they are unable to distinguish between their production or because the categories the signs describe are not clear enough. It is also conceivable that previous teaching employing the use of praise and other general forms of reward with many different signs has unlearned a 'natural' tendency to perceive and use signs differently.

Signs for proper names

An environment consists not only of events and activities but also of people. It is often difficult to find good ways to teach people's names, because the actual use of such names has few immediate consequences. It may also be difficult for the individual to understand what these names mean. One solution to this may be to use proper names as signal signs. In nursery schools, schools, institutions and community units, changes in staff members are often important events. The individuals generally have their favourites, i.e. people to whom they become particularly attached. Owing to the nature of shift work in such institutions, it can be difficult to comprehend staff changes and it is often a problem for the individuals to know which members of staff are present. Staff changes often take place without the disabled individuals' knowledge, which makes it difficult for them to have a complete grasp of the situation and increases their feelings of uncertainty and confusion. The absence of a particular staff member whom an individual expects to be present may, for example, be perceived as punishment if the absence is felt to be due to an event that occurred previously. For many autistic individuals, the inability to anticipate events and to have an idea of what is going to happen often leads to panic reactions. Using peoples' names as signal signs ensures that individuals with communication disorders are always kept informed about which members of staff are present. This may increase the likelihood of communicative initiative on the part of the individual.

In practical terms this may be done by members of staff informing everyone individually that they have arrived. For an individual who uses manual signs, this is done by the

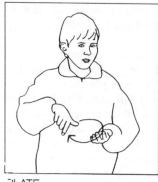

PLATE

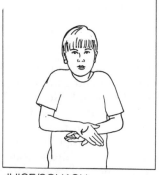

JUICE/SQUASH

member of staff guiding the individual's hands to sign the name. Each staff member should have his or her own sign. The name sign may be the first letter in the staff member's name using the hand alphabet, as is usual when presenting oneself to deaf people who use sign language, or it may be a constructed sign. If graphic signs are used, the name sign could be a drawing or a photograph of the person, at which the individual is guided to point. For individuals with somewhat more developed language skills, it may be sufficient to show them the picture or perform the manual sign. At a later stage the same signs or pictures could be used to talk about the people.

Expanding use

Expanding the use of signs is in many ways as important as expanding the sign vocabulary. Expanding use means using one particular sign about several different exemplars of the same object, several performances of the same activity, in several different situations and in connection with various other signs. When training expanded use, the object or activity being trained is varied systematically. The sign PLATE can be used to refer to large and small plates, as well as different coloured plates. For example, when practising the sign SQUASH, the situation may be varied by using different glasses and cups.

A significant feature of expanded use is that the signs are used in new ways. When the individual seems to have understood how to use a sign to obtain something, naming should be introduced. Practising naming is often linked to the act of responding to the sign WHAT, i.e. 'What is that?'. This skill is not particularly functional in itself, but the aim is that the naming will acquire a social function. Commenting about something without wanting it is a fairly advanced skill, but the individuals and adults in contact with them may enjoy sitting together naming objects, activities and pictures. It may be difficult to design situations that are appropriate for commentary, but unusual and funny situations are suitable.

> Billy is a severely handicapped 3-year-old boy. He was taught to name a ball but showed no interest in the task. One day a helper crept behind the teacher, who sat opposite Billy, held a large ball above the teacher's head and pretended she was going to drop it. When Billy saw this, he pointed excitedly at the teacher and vocalised what sounded like ball (Halle, Alpert and Anderson, 1984).

One of the main aims of teaching naming is that the number of signs the individual uses to obtain something will increase without special training. Naming is therefore a

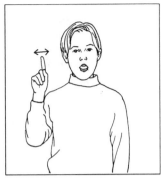

WHAT

more economical way of training new signs. Both this and the desire that naming be used to comment on events implies that naming should not unilaterally be linked to the conversational partners' WHAT. The signs should be able to be used to answer different approaches. WHAT is also a useful sign that allows the individual to learn the name of an object or activity and to get comments on activities that are taking place. It is therefore essential that the teacher and the individual take turns at naming and asking questions in the teaching situations.

> Andrew is out for a walk with his teacher. A helicopter flies overhead. Andrew points at the helicopter and signs WHAT. The teacher shows him how to sign HELICOPTER.

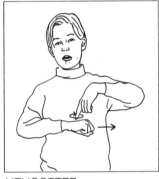

HELICOPTER

Situations that begin with an individual signing WHAT generally produce good conditions for teaching. The situation is initiated by the individuals themselves, based on a wish to gain information about an event or activity. Both the individual and the conversational partner focus on the same object or event, and the individual is interested and motivated to learn new signs. By using the sign WHAT, the individual will also be able to obtain information about *new* interests. Thus, using the sign WHAT will gradually lead to a more user-controlled choice of signs. In the case of individuals who occasionally ask the names of new objects or activities, it is a good idea to have a sign dictionary (e.g. *Communication Link: A Dictionary of Signs* – Smith, 1988) available whenever possible. Likewise, one should try to have as many graphic signs available at all times as is practically possible.

Sign dictionary

A personal sign dictionary should be made for the individual as soon as the sign teaching is initiated. In the sign dictionary the translation of each sign should be noted alphabetically, as well as which signs are being trained, and which are being used, understood, or both. The book should also contain a description or drawing of how a manual sign is ordinarily performed, and how the individual performs it. In the case of graphic signs, the dictionary should contain a description of how the individual points, and whether combinations of signs are used to express specific words that are not on the board. With the help of the sign dictionary, anyone who is in contact with the individual can quickly get an idea of the signs that are used and understood. If the sign vocabulary and number of sign sentences grows large, the sign dictionary will also be an aid to keeping account of which signs have been learned.

The sign dictionary represents a way of discovering new ideas for expanding sign use. For example, one may look at the activity signs in the sign dictionary and try to find object signs that can be used in connection with these activities. Conversely, one may look at the object signs in order to find activities where these object signs can be used. Both of these approaches are examples of a domain-oriented strategy. The dictionary will also makes it easier to ascertain whether there is anything the individual may need but does not know the sign for.

The sign dictionary is not only useful for the people in contact with the individuals. The individuals themselves will also draw benefit from it, and where possible the dictionary should be made together with the individual. It may be divided into domains, or some other system may be utilised that makes it easy for someone who is unable to read to find things. The sign dictionary becomes a type of reader, which the individual can be proud of. Since the words are listed together with the signs, it is also practical when an individual is with people who do not know signs.

Multiple sign utterances

Choosing signs and encouraging individuals to use multiple sign utterances are closely linked. Some signs are better suited than others to being combined to form multiple sign utterances, and these signs may help the user both to acquire new signs and to combine several signs to form utterances. In the early stages of normal language development, certain words are frequently used and are often combined with other words. Such words are called *pivots* (Braine, 1963). Once the individual has learned a number of signs, it is important to find signs than can function as pivots and encourage a natural sign acquisition without the need for special training.

Pivots may be activity signs that are combined with several objects, e.g. EAT APPLE, EAT BANANA, EAT BREAD. They may also be object signs that are used with a variety of activity signs, e.g. GET BALL, THROW BALL, ROLL BALL, KICK BALL. Signs such as GET, HAVE and GIVE are also suitable for use as pivots.

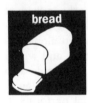

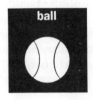

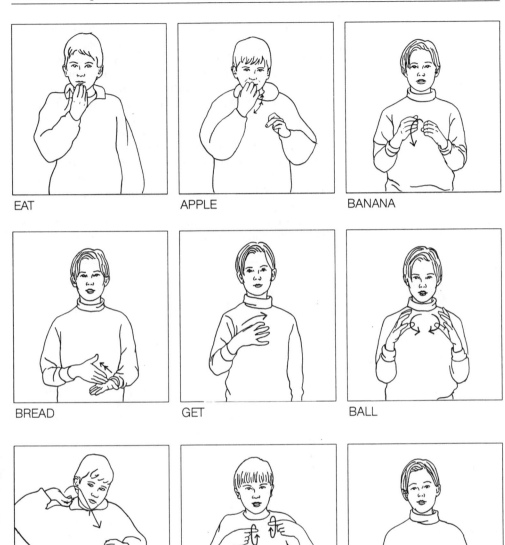

EAT   APPLE   BANANA

BREAD   GET   BALL

THROW   ROLL   GIVE

Sentences may also be produced by *chaining* certain expressive signs with more general signal signs. For example, OUT may be learned as a signal sign, and SWING and WALK as expressive signs. These can be combined as a means of informing an individual that he is going OUT WALK or OUT SWING. Later on the use of OUT may be expanded to include OUT SHOP and OUT VISIT. Utterances can be expanded beyond two signs by adding more links, e.g. OUT CAR SHOP, OUT PLAY SWING and OUT VISIT GRANDMOTHER. The signs in the sentences should be produced with the individuals' hands if they have not already demonstrated that they are capable of learning by observing other people using signs.

Signs that can be combined with more than one activity sign in the same way as OUT, as well as signs that can be

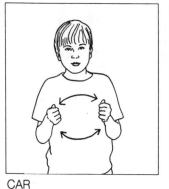

CAR

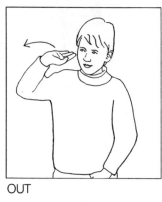

OUT

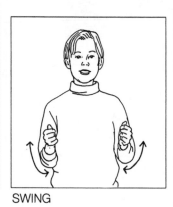

SWING

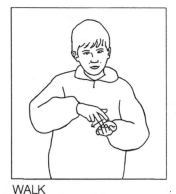

WALK

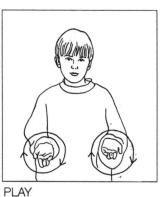

PLAY

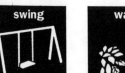

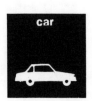

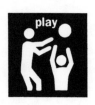

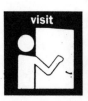

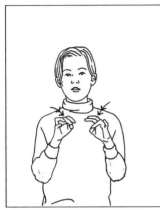

FINISHED

combined with more than one object sign, are well suited to expanding an individual's sign vocabulary. FINISHED can easily be combined with an activity sign, e.g. FINISHED WORK. Command signs may also be used in sentences, e.g. FETCH CASSETTE, FETCH MINERAL WATER. With a little imagination, together with knowledge of the individual's interests and likes, this approach may be used in expressive training. The teacher and the individual can take turns at giving instructions, so that the teacher sometimes has to fetch the mineral water or cassette. Such utterances may also be used as a means of talking about events, often in combination with the name of one of the staff members or other residents: PETER GET TRAIN RAILS, MARY FINISHED MINERAL WATER.

Part of the aim of using sentences is that the individuals

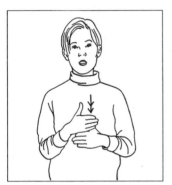

WORK

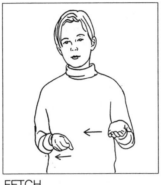

FETCH

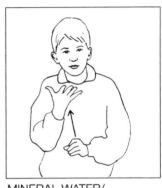

MINERAL WATER/
FIZZY DRINK

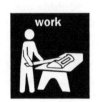

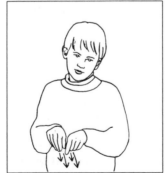

RAILS

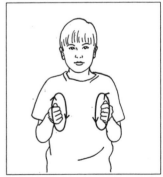

TRAIN

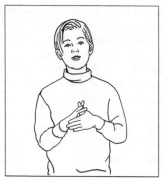

FIRST

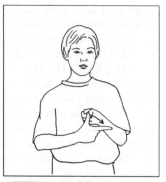

AFTERWARDS/THEN

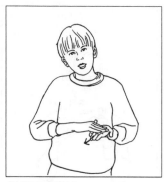

CLEAN/TIDY

will learn to communicate about sequences of activities and activities that are not taking place at the time of conversation, or objects that are not visible. This will enable them to obtain objects that are not present in the situation or suggest activities that are currently not taking place, specify to a greater extent what it is they want, and give them a better grasp of what is going to happen. It is often difficult for mentally handicapped or autistic people to understand the order of events that will take place. In such instances it is worth teaching the signs FIRST–THEN as a sentence construction. The individual may then be told FIRST TIDY, THEN WALK or FIRST MUSIC, THEN SPORT.

As sign vocabulary and sentence use expand, it becomes possible to combine more and more signs, and in general the sentences produced will resemble those found among children with normal language development (Fulwiler and Fouts, 1976). The sentences will contain object signs and activity signs, as well as signs for qualities such as LARGE, SMALL and RED, and prepositions such as ABOVE, UNDER and IN. Many of these sentence constructions are easy to train in ordinary classroom situations, but it is essential that part of the teaching takes place in other environments. Even when such a high linguistic level has been reached, signs to be introduced should be chosen on the basis of assumptions about which signs will best contribute to improve the individuals' overall situation.

Although many of the sentences will resemble sentences found among people with normal language development, the individuals will also have idiosyncratic sign combinations that are not easily understood by those who do not know them. Each individual's sign dictionary should also contain this kind of sentence.

Computer-based aids enable users of graphic signs to use one sign to produce ready-made sentences. This may

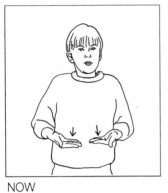

NOW

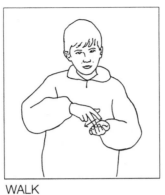

WALK

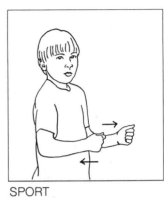

SPORT

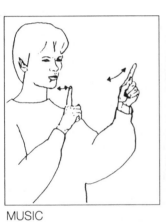

MUSIC

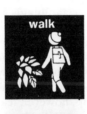

walk

music

large

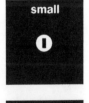

small

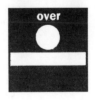

over

under

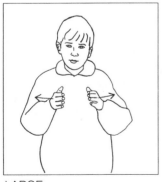

LARGE

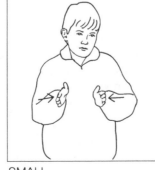

SMALL

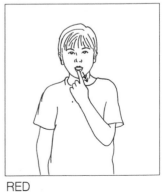

RED

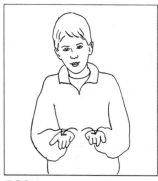

BOOK

seem practical, since the communication then bears a closer resemblance to normal communication, but as long as the individual is in an early stage of language development, the use of ready-made sentences is not recommended. Single words may be interpreted in more ways than a sentence and will therefore provide more communicative opportunities. For example, BOOK may mean 'There is the book', 'Take the book away' or 'Give me the book'. *Give me the book* has only one meaning. The strategies for combining signs to form sentences are also based on single words, and the use of ready-made sentences may hinder the individual's learning of the sentence-making process.

The expressive language group

The expressive language group is very heterogeneous group. In cases where the major problem is a lack of expressive means, it may be necessary to employ some of the methods discussed above. Other individuals who belong to this group may have normal intellectual skills or a moderate degree of mental handicap. For the expressive language group, however, learning difficulties do not necessarily impede an individual's ability to learn to communicate. The limitations lie in the individual's lack of speech and the demands made on the individual's motor functions by the design of the aid.

Here the focus is on individuals with good language comprehension and a substantial vocabulary. Exactly what is implied by 'substantial' is hard to say, but around 1000 signs or more is a reasonable estimate. This is not a large vocabulary; 2–3-year-old children have a vocabulary of at least this many words. However, it is rare to find such a large vocabulary among users of communication aids who have not learned to write. The sign vocabulary of children between 5 and 12 years old usually consists of 100–350 signs.

User involvement

For people with a good understanding of language who learn to express themselves with the aid of graphic signs, the fact that one sign is chosen at the expense of another represents a considerable barrier to social participation. The sign vocabulary determines which subjects can be discussed and which conversations are possible. Today it is constantly repeated that the signs on a communication board should be chosen on the basis of what is useful for users in their particular environment. However, in many instances too much emphasis is given to signs for care, nursing, etc., despite the fact that individuals themselves seldom talks of these things (Beukelman and Yorkston, 1984). The individuals need signs that can be used in a large variety of situations, signs that reflect their interests and make it possible for them to converse about a great number of subjects.

It is usually professionals who decide which signs individuals have on their communication boards. To make sure that the signs will be useful, it is essential that the users are involved as much as possible when signs are being selected. User involvement in the sign selection process is especially important for older children, adolescents and adults but attempts should be made to involve the users at the earliest possible stage. This may be done by examining situations in which the children usually participate or would like to participate, radio and television programmes, the dictionary of the graphic sign system they use, other lists of signs, ordinary dictionaries and books that have recently been read to the children. Thereafter the children and the adult helpers can discuss the words and the situations in which they could be used. At the same time, a discussion of this type will give teachers considerable insight into the children's language comprehension and life situation, as well as providing clues as to how conditions could be made more favourable for the individuals. As far as possible the children should be allowed to choose the signs for themselves. If there are signs the adults believes to be important for the children, these can be presented in another context, perhaps with the phrase: *I have a useful word for you*.

Expanding situations where signs may be used

Many individuals who belong to the expressive language group are severely motor impaired. They have limited mobility, and thus acquire a narrower experience of life than their peers. In order to expand sign use, they must be given the opportunity to participate in a variety of different situations. Nursery school and school form an extremely important part of the environment in which all children grow up, but this is perhaps even more so in the case of motor-impaired children and adolescents, who are less able to participate in leisure-time and outdoor activities. The teaching of communication use is often scholastic, and planned with the requirements of nursery school and school in mind. Professionals should free themselves from these restrictions and expand the individual's situational repertoire. This is not an easy task, and challenges one's powers of innovation and imagination. Helpers, brothers and sisters and peers can play an important role in expanding participation in different situations and help by making conditions more favourable for expansion.

For an expanded environment to lead to expanded understanding and use of signs, individuals must have access to their means of communication whenever it is needed. Access to communication aids is often poor outside school and special teaching situations. Many children and adolescents who sit in a pushchair or wheelchair have their communication board placed behind them in a carrier. This means that the adult helpers control when conversations may take place. They may take the communication board out when they themselves wish to communicate, or when they believe the child or youth has something to say.

One of the difficulties with using communication aids is that it is not always easy to point at them with the hand or in other ways in situations where there would otherwise be a good deal of communication. This applies for example during washing, mealtimes, in the car and in bed. Eye-pointing may be an alternative, but there must be sufficient space between each of the signs and they must be placed so that it is possible to follow the individual's direction of gaze without misunderstanding. One way of solving this may be for the conversational partner to wear a waistcoat with signs on, so that the individual can point with his eyes or select signs by means of dependent scanning, i.e. the conversational partner points at the signs and the individual confirms when he or she is pointing at the correct sign (Figure 33). However, communication boards should, if possible, be fixed and not move with the conversational partner.

Figure 33. A vest can be used as a communication board.

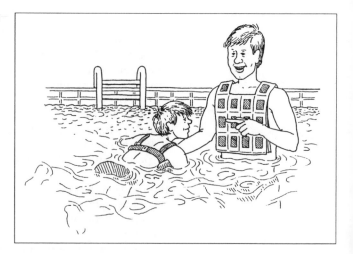

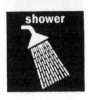

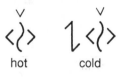

Mealtimes and care

Even people with communication boards that are suitably placed will as a rule be unable to communicate in the bath, in the toilet, during mealtimes (with the exception of choosing between types of food), in bed, etc. It is important that the individuals are able to communicate in these situations, because individuals with motor impairment generally spend a long time over meals and care. Conversations during mealtimes also quickly become meaningless because they are generally about food, i.e. what the individual wants to eat or drink. There is usually little to be said about this since there are few choices that need to be made during the course of a normal mealtime. The contrast to other people's conversations is great. Other children talk mostly about what they have done or are thinking of doing, and spend very little time discussing the food. In order to facilitate conversation during mealtimes, a number of fixed signs may be placed where the child usually sits, fastened so that they do not end up under the plate or otherwise concealed. It is also a good idea to have a number of domain signs easily available, for use when more specialised subjects arise.

It is not so easy to take a communication board into the bathroom, but PIC signs, Blissymbols or words may be put on the bathroom wall. These should include words that pertain to and are important in that particular situation. For very small children, this may be a picture of a bath toy they are fond of, for somewhat older children and adults the signs HOT, COLD, MORE and SHOWER are important so that they may say how they experience the situation, and whether it should be changed. In this situation too, though, it is a good idea to have something else to talk about, especially if the individual is fond of bathing and does so often. Care is time-consuming, and it is advantageous if the individual has the opportunity to communicate, even though this means that the care takes even longer. Individuals with extensive motor impairments also benefit from the presence of signs that are used to indicate the way other people handle them. Such signs enable individuals to instruct people who do not know them very well. When the individuals have access to signs that make it easier for other people to adjust, the adjustment will come naturally because the helpers will be more sensitive and expect instruction. This will help improve the general situation (cf. Dalhoff, 1986; Hagen, Porter and Brink, 1973).

In the car

Communication in a car is often difficult because the driver has to keep his or her eyes on the road and because jolts and turns make pointing imprecise. At the same time there is plenty to see, and many situations that lend themselves to comment. Number plates, reckless drivers and road-hogs are often objects of attention for children. It is not so easy to give the individual access to a large vocabulary, but the situation can be made considerably more *active* and interesting if there are a few signs available. The user of a communication aid may be the 'navigator' and say RIGHT, LEFT, and STRAIGHT AHEAD at junctions if the car journey follows a familiar route. RIGHT, LEFT, BEHIND and AHEAD may be used to indicate the location of points of interest. Synthetic or digitised speech may relieve some of the communication problems. (Technical aids can be attached to the lighter socket in the car.) If there are several people in the car, dependent scanning may be utilised, perhaps by reading aloud (auditory scanning) if the seating arrangements make it difficult to see the board. If there is a specific destination, or the route passes particularly interesting places, it may provide a good opportunity to introduce new signs, which the adult then uses to support his or her own comments. One may also stop from time to time if there is anything that should be looked at or talked about. If several children with communication aids are on a trip together, the adult can relay the conversations between them.

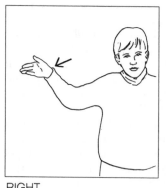
RIGHT

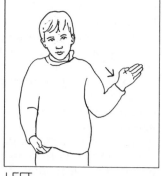
LEFT

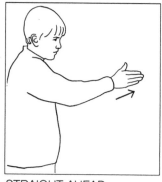
STRAIGHT AHEAD

behind in front

In bed and at night

Many disabled people need help to get into or out of bed. They are also frequently ill and spend time in bed, so it is important that they have the opportunity to communicate in the bedroom. The bedroom is often the place where children are cuddled and hear small talk. Fairy-tales may be read aloud, and the children and their caregivers can talk about what is happening in them. This activity, along with other types of conversation, helps to provide disabled children with the same cultural base around which other children's activities are built.

On occasions it can be very important for children to be able to communicate at night. The reason a child cries and is restless may simply be that he or she is thirsty, and if the child can say so and is given something to drink, everyone will get to sleep. But a child may also cry because of a nightmare or an ailment. It may take the parents a long time to find out what is wrong, which will result in a lack of sleep and perhaps grumpiness the next morning. A few graphic signs on the wall or a stand beside the bed may help reduce the number of sleepless nights and make the child feel more secure.

Increased access to signs

The actual design of the communication board and the number of words it can contain will depend on the method of pointing or scanning and the user's motor skills. If direct selection is utilised, it is important that the signs are not so small that it becomes easy to misunderstand which sign the user is pointing at. Since there is a limit to the number of signs that can be placed on a surface, the vocabulary should at all times be best suited to the user's needs. This implies, among other things, that the teacher or caregiver may have to swap signs instead of just adding new ones, and that it may be necessary to have more than one board.

There has been virtually no research into the effects different vocabularies have on language development. Carlson (1981) mentions that a child who did not use the communication board began to use it when the vocabulary was changed. However, with the exception of how 'useful' it is, little is known about how a vocabulary should best be worked out to encourage the development of communication skills and competence. There is every reason to believe, though, that giving emphasis to a general vocabulary, i.e. a *surface-oriented* expansion of vocabulary, will reinforce the lack of communicative initiative and limited conversational skills. Using a domain-oriented strategy when developing vocabulary makes it easier for individuals to say something new, and thus helps them to make their own contributions to the conversation and continue it in such a way that the conversational partner does not lose interest.

In the discussion of communication boards, emphasis has often been given to the fact that a small number of words constitute a large part of what is said. This has been used as fuel for arguments stressing that it is possible to communicate effectively with a small number of words, which is true as long as the conversation is kept on a very superficial level. At the same time there has been a strong focus on signs that provide individuals with the opportunity to express fundamental needs in everyday life. If the individuals are to have a chance of conversing on anything other than a superficial level and expressing anything more than basic needs, their vocabulary must be adapted to fit the situation at hand. Increasing the vocabulary alone is not a suitable method of developing conversational skills, since the users will almost immediately become dependent on conversational partners to formulate questions and comments.

There are a number of reasons why reorganising an individual's sign vocabulary requires swapping words. If new signs were added all the time, then the vocabulary would become too large, even if some of the signs were transferred to other boards. The vocabulary a conversational partner sees plays an important role in assessing an individual, and determines which subjects will be discussed and how the conversation will start. Conversational partners tend to treat users of communication aids as though they are younger than they actually are (Shane and Cohen, 1981). If the words on the communication board are childish, this tendency will be reinforced. Words that are too childish should be replaced. For example, the picture of a teddy-bear on a child's board should be removed once the child becomes older.

Even when the user has several boards, there will be clear limits to how large the vocabulary can grow. One main communication board and its sub-boards, and any sub-sub-boards, in principle constitute a tree-like structure. Using several boards makes it difficult to keep account of the vocabulary, and in time becomes impractical. Computer technology may relieve this problem, since the boards do not take up so much physical space. If an individual is able to choose between four signs three times, this gives a vocabulary of 64 words (Figure 34). Three levels with 16 signs on each page give the individual access to 4096 signs (16 x 16 x 16). An individual with a reasonable degree of dexterity should be able to reach each sign quickly, but an

Figure 34. *Search structure when choosing between four signs.*

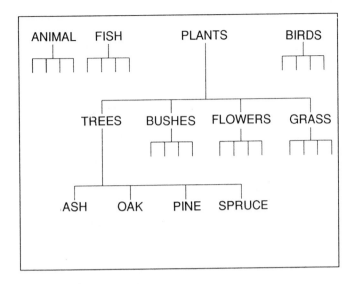

individual with more extensive motor difficulties will take considerably longer to reach each one. However, the main problem is to organise the signs so that the individual is able to remember the position at any given time without any form of visual support other than the view of the communication board displayed on the screen. There will be a total of 256 different screens (16 x 16) in a search structure with three levels of 16 signs each.

Building vocabularies in communication aids is a field where there has been little research. The sign structure in a technical aid should be designed so that the individual is able to grow with it. It should be able to retain those skills that are developed and build upon them. A tree structure is not the only conceivable form of search structure. One system that utilises some of the potential provided by technology is Minspeak (Baker, 1986). Basically, it is a coding system for sentences, which are spoken with the aid of synthetic or digitised speech. By pressing keys in different orders, different sentences can be produced. For example, if the keys MILK+HOT are pressed, the machine may say *I want hot milk*, but *The milk is too hot* if the key combination HOT+MILK is used. Which key combination will correspond to which sentence is determined in advance. It is also possible to have several topics, so that the sentence that is spoken is dependent on both the topic that is chosen and the order in which the keys are pressed. Minspeak is not dependent on any specific graphic sign system. In fact, Baker (1986) argues in favour of signs that are unique to the individual because he believes that one's own associations are easier to remember than sign systems constructed by others. However, it may be an advantage to use an

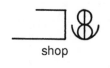

shop

baby   car

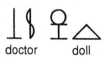

doctor   doll

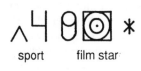

sport   film star

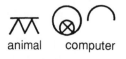

animal   computer

stamp

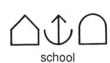

school

history   mathematics

work

ordinary sign system because it is easier to use it without the coded sentences if the batteries run down or the machine develops a fault.

When describing the individual's everyday situation, the teacher should try to find central *domains* that will promote more profound conversation. For younger children, domain signs such as SHOP, BABY, CAR, DOCTOR and DOLL may be used in conjunction with role playing and games. Older children and adolescents may use signs connected with special interests such as SPORT, POP MUSIC, FILM STARS, ANIMALS, COMPUTERS, STAMPS and BOOKS, or vocabulary associated with SCHOOL (HISTORY, MATHEMATICS, GEOGRAPHY, etc.) or WORK. More general, single boards may also be adapted to specific environments. The vocabularies used may differ somewhat at home, school, in the youth club, on the street, etc. When producing such domain- and situation-dependent boards, words the individual knows and unfamiliar words may both be included, so that the board helps to develop the individual's vocabulary. The boards should be reviewed systematically and revised regularly, e.g. four times a year, so that the individual is not unnecessarily restricted by the existing vocabulary.

The introduction of domain boards may have a positive effect on the environment and on professionals who will be forced to design situations that suit the vocabulary. In this way it is more likely that the individual will acquire a greater variety of linguistic experiences. Adults, as well as other children and adolescents who see the new communication boards, will perhaps begin to discuss new subjects when they converse with the aided speaker. An exciting domain board may make more people want to initiate conversations.

Expanding the vocabulary by using sign combinations

When a communication aid user with a limited vocabulary does not have a sign for the word that is wanted, he or she must find other ways of expressing that word. For example, in order to say something about chess an individual may perhaps point at the signs GAME and SQUARE. This sign combination could just as easily be interpreted as 'cards', 'ludo' or 'checkers' if none of these signs appeared on the communication board either. The individual might then be obliged to give the conversational partner several more clues before he or she understood. This paraphrasing is called *analogy*.

Blissymbols are built up as a system of analogies. In principle it should be possible for the user to construct any word freely from the basic Blissymbols, but some analogies

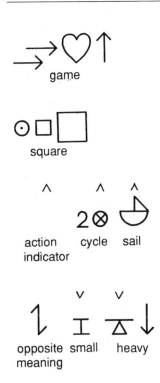

game

square

action   cycle   sail
indicator

opposite small   heavy
meaning

large   light

have been established by the International Bliss Committee. Using analogies makes it difficult to estimate the real size of the vocabulary of a user of an aid that uses the Blissymbols or other systems in which the signs are easy to combine. In the Bliss system combinations with ACTION change a noun into a verb. ACTION + BICYCLE becomes TO CYCLE, ACTION + SAILBOAT becomes TO SAIL. Combining a sign with OPPOSITE-MEANING produces an antonym. Thus, OPPOSITE-MEANING + LARGE means SMALL, OPPOSITE-MEANING + HEAVY means LIGHT. However, this method of expressing concepts also exists in the language of children without such combinations being regarded as separate words. When testing young children with ITPA, it is not uncommon to receive the answer *Not heavy* to the question *Lead is heavy, feathers are ...?*

Analogies are primarily associated with Blissymbols since this system is explicitly based on analogy. However, it is also common to find analogies in Rebus (Figure 35), and in principle the signs in all graphic sign systems may be combined to form new words. This applies also to script when the user has limited spelling skills, or when it is quicker to use a combination of words by analogy rather than spelling out a long word. The PIC signs HOUSE + SPORT may mean GYMNASIUM. HOUSE + LETTER may mean POST OFFICE if there are otherwise no signs to express these concepts (Figure 35).

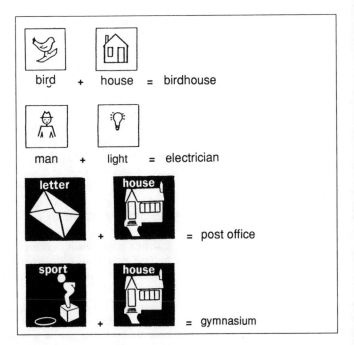

bird + house = birdhouse

man + light = electrician

letter + house = post office

sport + house = gymnasium

Figure 35. *Combinations of Rebus signs and PIC signs.*

The use of analogies places considerable demands on both the user and the listener. The user must have an idea of what the listener is able to understand, while the listener must have both a good imagination and a good deal of empathy in order to understand what it is the user is trying to say. Even relatively uncomplicated statements are sometimes difficult to communicate. The use of analogies therefore assumes that those who will use and understand the systems receive the correct teaching. Recent teaching has placed too much emphasis on ready-made sign combinations and combinations using grammatical signs, such as OPPOSITE, PLURAL and ACTION. The users should learn to use the system in such a way so that the conversational partners need not have prior knowledge of the construction in order to understand what is being said. The best way of doing this is probably to use technical communication aids with the maximum number of combinations, where the word either appears on screen or is spoken artificially. Most graphic sign users who have a need for an extensive vocabulary are severely motor impaired, and it may therefore be possible to attach the aid to their wheelchairs.

From graphic signs to script

Vocabulary gradually ceases to be a problem for those individuals who learn to read and write, but most of them will need signs at least until they reach the age of 7 or 8. Many motor-impaired individuals learn to read at a later stage, or never achieve functional reading skills. Both for those who learn to read and for those who do not, it is important that as many of the words they need as possible are made available to them at an early stage. It should also be possible to expand the vocabulary as is the case in normal language development. For those who do not learn to read or who learn to read at a later stage, it is crucial that they get access to knowledge in other ways than through reading, so that they are not unnecessarily hindered in areas in which they have a generally good basis.

There is a close link between problems of articulation and reading and writing difficulties. Reading and writing difficulties often occur among people with paralysis of the mouth, larynx and pharynx. It is not known what distinguishes good readers from bad ones, but there is reason to believe that both individual differences and the teaching of reading skills are of importance (Morley, 1972; Smith et al., 1989).

Sometimes the teaching is begun too late and makes slow progress. For children who are unable to talk but are nonetheless able to use a normal keyboard or concept keyboard, it is worthwhile trying to give them access to synthetic speech at an early stage. There is no reason why these children should not be able to learn to 'speak' in this way as long as this is not used in connection with traditional reading teaching. They can use the machine to 'babble' and to find words. The machine should be available at all times so that the children can practise using words in the same way as children who learn to speak normally (cf. Weir, 1966).

A similar approach may be a good alternative to traditional reading teaching. Instead of learning to read, the child learns to write. With the aid of synthetic speech, a computer pronounces what the individual has written. People with reading and writing difficulties do not usually have great problems recognising spoken words. Thus, the computer performs what the speech-impaired individual finds most difficult – articulating words or sequences of letters. The individual can learn to write because the feedback received from the computer's speech forms the basis of a correction of spelling mistakes and ascertaining the correct spelling. This technology may be combined with programs that check spelling so that words like *near* and *build* are not written *n-e-r-e* and *b-i-l-d*.

As yet there has been little systematic research into the use of synthetic speech in reading teaching. However, some studies indicate that such an approach may yield positive results (Koke and Neilson, 1987).

There are also examples where children who have been able to read have been given boards containing Blissymbols, and that teaching in the use of Blissymbols has been favoured instead of reading teaching (Smith et al., 1989). This is probably due to the fact that many professionals seem to believe that the graphic signs, for example in the Blissymbol system, express more than just their gloss. Thus, they feel that it is more meaningful to combine ANIMAL+LONG+NOSE to form ELEPHANT than *animal+long+nose* to produce *elephant*. This is of course incorrect.

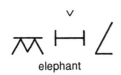
elephant

One can just as well form analogies with script as with Blissymbols. The person who interprets an utterance in Blissymbols does anyway combine the glosses as they are written above the signs. Although it is easier for children who are unable to read to learn Blissymbols rather than normal script, once they have learned to spell they will find it easier to read script rather than Blissymbols.

Both Blissymbols and Rebus use letters as a part of the sign system. Single letters are used actively to give words different meanings, as in the example with the sign CAT. However, there are no ready-made procedures or teaching strategies that deal with the transition from Blissymbols to

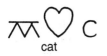
cat

script. This is a serious flaw because many individuals use Blissymbols when they begin to learn to read. It also means that the Blissymbols are not being used to develop language skills in the best way possible. The acquisition of reading skills may be delayed or hindered. Rebus signs are better suited to the development of reading skills. It may be useful to adopt some of the strategies used in the Rebus sign system, and perhaps utilise them in conjunction with Blissymbols.

Strategies used with Blissymbols are not the most effective for individuals who are able to write.

> Alan is a 20-year-old motor-impaired man. He has a good understanding of language and also has good writing skills. He uses a board with both Blissymbols and letters. When he wants to say 'cow', he points first at the sign ANIMAL and then spells out the word *c-o-w*.

For people who use script as their main form of communication, with the linguistic freedom it provides, it is necessary to acquire those strategies that are best suited to the communication form they use. Many Blissymbols have short glosses. For the individual who is able to spell, it may be useful to have a number of ready-made words and phrases so that the communication process requires less time. It is not the short words that need to be replaced by analogies, but rather the long words that occur relatively often. A decision should be made as to which words these are, but it is clear that it will not apply to all the signs generally found on boards containing Blissymbols.

Ready-made vocabularies

There is a tendency among professionals to suggest the same words for different people, without taking into account differences in terms of age, interests and the individual's general situation. It is rare that professionals sit down and take their time discussing which words should be chosen with the parents, brothers and sisters, and others who know the individual well.

There are a number of ready-made vocabularies available for use by individuals who are taught augmentative communication or given other forms of language training. These vocabularies vary in size. Some of them are intended to be used explicitly with a specific sign system, while others are intended as general guidelines, independent of whether the individual is receiving teaching in speech, script, manual signs or graphic sign systems.

Two vocabularies that are supposedly suitable for use with children, and which have a central place in the litera-

Table 4. *The words suggested by Fristoe and Lloyd (1980)(F&L) and the first two stages of the Norwegian Makaton (Walker and Ekeland, 1985)(W&E).* ture, are shown in Table 4. There are approximately 80 words in each, and they are intended to be used as the individuals' *first words.* Makaton (Walker and Ekeland, 1985) consists of nine stages. Only the first two stages are included here, since they contain approximately the same number of words as the vocabulary suggested by Fristoe and Lloyd

Substantive words

	W&E	F&L		W&E	F&L
APPLE		X	POTTY		X
BABY		X	SCHOOL		X
BALL	X	X	SHIRT		X
BATHROOM		X	SHOES		X
BED	X		SISTER	X	
BIRD	X	X	SOCKS		X
BISCUIT	X		SPOON	X	X
BOOK	X	X	STAFF	X	
BOY	X		SWEETS	X	
BREAD	X		SUGAR	X	
BRICKS	X		TABLE	X	X
BROTHER	X		TEDDY	X	
BUTTER	X		TELEVISION	X	X
CAKE	X	X	TOILET	X	X
CANDY		X	TREE	X	
CAR	X	X	TROUSERS		X
CASSETTE PLAYER	X	X	WATER		X
CAT	X	X	WINDOW	X	X
CHAIR	X	X	YOU	X	X
CHEESE	X				
COAT		X			
COFFEE	X				
COMB		X			
CUP	X	X			
DADDY	X				
DOG	X	X			
DOLL	X				
DOOR	X	X			
DRINK		X			
EGG	X				
FATHER		X			
FIRE (HEATING)	X				
FLOWER	X				
FOOD	X	X			
FORK	X				
GIRL	X	X			
HAT		X			
HOME	X				
HOUSE	X	X			
I		X			
ICE CREAM	X				
JAM	X				
KNIFE	X				
LADY	X				
LAMP	X				
LIGHT	X				
MAN	X				
MILK	X	X			
MUMMY/MOTHER	X	X			
(Name signs)		X			
PLATE	X				

Relational words

	W&E	F&L
AND	X	
BAD	X	X
BATH	X	
BIG/LARGE		X
BROKEN		X
CLEAN	X	
COLD	X	
COME	X	
DIRTY	X	X
DOWN		X
DRINK	X	X
EAT	X	X
FALL		X
GET		X
GIVE	X	X
GONE		X
GOOD MORNING	X	
GOOD	X	X
GOODBYE	X	
HAPPY		X
HEAVY		X
HELP		X
HERE	X	
HOT	X	X
KISS		X
LEAVE	X	X
LIE DOWN		X
LOOK/WATCH	X	X
MAKE		X
MORE		X
NOT	X	
NO	X	X
OPEN		X
PLAY		X
RUN		X
SHOWER	X	
SIT		X
SLEEP	X	
STAND		X
STAND-UP	X	
STOP		X
THANK YOU	X	
THERE	X	
THIS/THAT/THOSE		X
THROW		X
UP		X
WALK		X
WASH	X	X
WHAT	X	
WHERE	X	
YES	X	

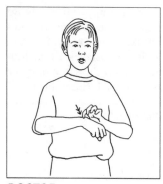

DOCTOR

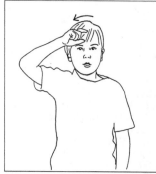

NURSE

(1980). Makaton is specifically intended to be used by small children, and is based, among other things, on studies of early language development. The second vocabulary is aimed especially at school-aged children (Fristoe and Lloyd, 1980). In some instances the lists have also been used with children and adults with well-developed comprehension skills. In the sign vocabularies no distinction is made between comprehension signs and expressive signs.

Since the lists are general, it is impossible to take into account the special characteristics of each individual child. Fristoe and Lloyd take care to say that the vocabulary is not suitable for everyone, but that many individuals will find it useful. On the other hand, Walker (1976) claims that the vocabulary in Makaton should be learned by everyone, although other words may be included as well. Her choice of words, stages and the teaching procedures that make up the Makaton vocabulary have met with considerable criticism (Byler, 1985; Kiernan et al., 1982).

A review of the two vocabularies shows how difficult it is to design a first vocabulary that many individuals will find useful, and demonstrates at the same time which criteria have been used in the selection process. There are many missing words that children might well need. On the other hand, the lists have many words associated with cleanliness and self-help, which the children themselves are rarely interested in using. Nor do older children, adolescents and adults use such signs particularly often, most likely because care/washing usually takes place at fixed times and without the individuals having any particular influence over the situation.

The vocabularies are divided into *substantive words* and *relational words*, in accordance with the suggestions of Lahey and Bloom (1977). Substantive words (nouns) include words that are used to indicate people, places or objects. Relational words are used to indicate relations

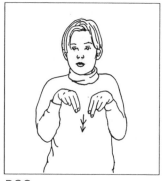

DOG

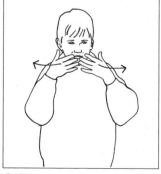

CAT

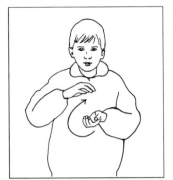

NAPPY

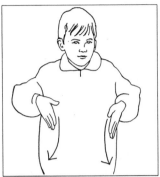

DRESS

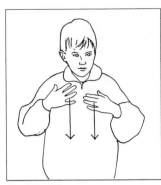

CLOTHES

between objects, and include such word classes as verbs, adjectives and prepositions.

Despite the fact that the vocabularies are designed with children in mind, there are few words for toys. Signs for animals may be useful for children who have a special interest in animals, or who have pets at home. HORSE could perhaps be used to signal riding, which is an activity enjoyed by many disabled individuals.

Signs for articles of clothing may be used as signal signs in a structured dressing setting. Surprisingly, Walker and Ekeland include no signs for clothes, while Fristoe and Lloyd include the most common. NAPPY is missing, as is DRESS. Signs for food items, fruit and sweets are among those signs that are first taught, because it is generally known what individuals like to eat. Walker and Ekeland include no fruit but, somewhat surprisingly, have chosen to include BUTTER. Fristoe and Lloyd include APPLE, but have no signs for other types of fruit or food. Neither of the vocabularies have the sign for ORANGE SQUASH or ORANGE JUICE, which are popular drinks. CHOCOLATE is also missing.

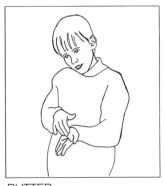

BUTTER

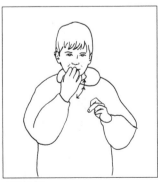

APPLE

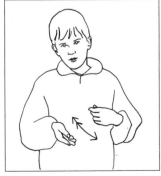

SUGAR

There are many names for eating utensils and household goods. The names of eating utensils may be useful. Walker and Ekeland include KNIFE, FORK and SPOON; Fristoe and Lloyd include only SPOON, and omit CUP and GLASS. Some of the signs for household goods may be used for naming without any clear functional objective. TELEVISION is a good expressive sign. Signs such as BED and TOILET are best suited as signal signs.

As a rule it is difficult to find good settings in which to teach signs for individuals. One possibility is to use them as signal signs. I, ME and YOU seem rather inappropriate since they are often implicit in the utterance.

Relational words are selected in order to be used together with many objects, and are not as contingent on the individual's interests and environment as is the case with many other words. GET, SEE, PLAY, HELP may be used in connection with many objects or activities and using them will facilitate the acquisition of new signs. Signs for specific activities are missing. Many of the signs may be of practical use when training self-help skills, and are thus suitable for use as signal signs. However, some of the signs seem to be rather unsuitable for a early functional vocabulary (e.g. CLEAN,

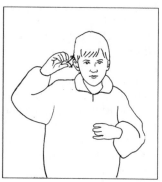

LAMP

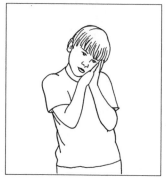

BED

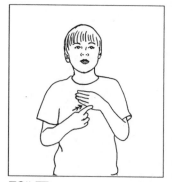

TOILET

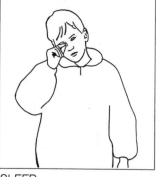

SLEEP

DIRTY, HERE, HOT, COLD, EVIL, HEAVY, UP, DOWN, AND, WHERE).

Walker and Ekeland include YES and NO. Using these signs in answer to questions is only meaningful if the individual is able to understand yes–no questions. This is a condition that many of those who receive teaching in augmentative communication do not fulfil. Moreover, YES and NO are dependent on the initiative of others. Fristoe and Lloyd do not use NO as an answer to a question but follow the arguments of Bloom and Lahey that NO may be used to express rejection, non-existence, the cessation of an action and in order to deny another person an activity. Rejection is something for which the majority of individuals who begin with augmentative communication already have an expression, which means it should be unnecessary to train them in this. As an indicator of non-existence, the word GONE is more suitable, since the sign NO will be used by others as a means of denying the individual an activity. STOP is better than NO when expressing the fact that an activity should cease. Nor is it easy to see how to design good teaching situations for rejection and non-existence. In general YES and NO are unsuitable in the early stages of teaching.

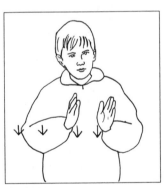

CLEAN

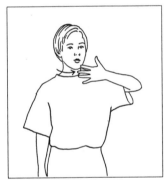

HOT

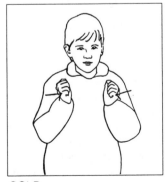

COLD

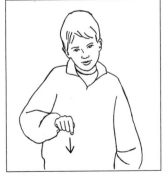

HERE

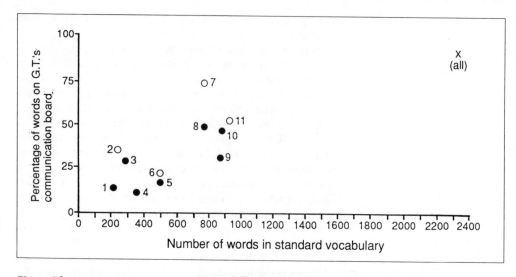

Figure 36. *Percentage of different vocabularies that a 36-year-old woman with cerebral palsy chose for her communication board. Her board contained 240 signs (Yorkston et al., 1989).*

How difficult it can be to find suitable signs in a ready-made vocabulary rather than taking the individual's own situation as a starting point is demonstrated in the following example (Yorkston et al., 1989).

G.T. was a 36-year-old woman with cerebral palsy who was unable to read and write. She had recently been given a board containing 24 Blissymbols. The board was in effect her first vocabulary, but her comprehension skills suggested that she needed a far larger vocabulary. She was given a communication aid that utilised synthetic speech, and she chose her vocabulary herself together with a team of professionals. Once she had begun to use a number of words, the team produced a description of her environment and a communication diary. Together with the team of professionals, G.T. also reviewed four standard vocabularies.

The total number of words on G.T.'s board was 240. Most of these words were of a general nature, chosen on the basis of their presumed frequency of use. Words that occurred infrequently were avoided. The selection of signs was thus in line with the needs that a standard vocabulary is supposed to meet. A comparison with 11 standard vocabularies showed that none of them contained all the 240 words on her board, even though some of the vocabularies were fairly extensive. Most of them covered well below 50 per cent of her words (Figure 36). Neither did the total of all the vocabularies – 2327 different words – cover her needs.

A lot of research time is spent on trying to find general vocabularies that are suitable for the task of augmentative communication teaching. This is a seemingly impossible task. However, together with other word lists, these vocabularies may constitute part of the material that will provide ideas for the production of a sign vocabulary suitable for an individual in need of augmentative communication.

Chapter 10
Conversational skills

Individuals who belong to the alternative, supportive and expressive language groups are all characterised by poor conversational skills. However, the differences between these groups in terms of language comprehension, social skills and interests are so great that objectives and methods utilised to encourage conversational skills differ greatly. Despite these differences, an improvement in conversational skills will lead to increased independence and a sense of belonging and equality. Most users of augmentative communication are dependent on others, both in order to perform daily tasks and in their leisure time. Conversation is a means of exchanging information and viewpoints and influencing others. Improving individuals' mastery of conversation makes it easier for them to make known their own wishes and viewpoints, influence others, express interests and make their own decisions.

In language development, conversations with adults imply training in language, concepts and values. Such conversations give the adults the opportunity to comment on what the children say and do, tell them the names of objects and activities, how particular objects are used, and explain to the children what they can and cannot do. For the children, conversations with adults form a significant part of the socialisation process. Children with extensive language and communication disorders, or children who have difficulty in expressing themselves due to motor impairments, miss out on a great deal of this type of natural learning. A central objective is therefore that the augmentative communication should compensate for the lack of learning opportunities caused by the disability.

A lack of conversational skills also has the negative effect that children and adults in need of augmentative communication derive few benefits from interaction with other people. The problems individuals in the expressive language group encounter in trying to say what they want to say are a daily source of frustration. Conversations become stereotypical and boring. For many of those who belong to the supportive language group, the experience of not being understood leads to shyness and embarrassment. For all three groups with users of augmentative communication, improving conversational skills may lead to increased intercourse with others and give the interaction a richer content.

Alternative language group

Traditionally, little attention has been paid to conversational skills when teaching language to people with language disorders. The main objective of augmentative communication teaching has been to teach individuals to use single signs as a means of obtaining something or naming an object or activity. The extent to which existing standardised teaching programmes actually promote the skills that enable individuals to converse is therefore unknown.

The basic conversational skills consist of starting a conversation and maintaining it, taking turns, changing topics, taking into account different conversational partners and repairing any interruptions in the conversation caused by misunderstandings or other reasons. These skills are difficult to acquire for autistic people, who belong to the alternative language group.

Keeping a long conversation going often proves to be a major problem, and it is extremely difficult to get autistic and severely disabled people to make independent contributions to conversations. Typically, a dialogue will consist of only two utterances if it is the individual who starts the dialogue, or three if it is the conversational partner who

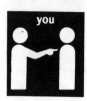

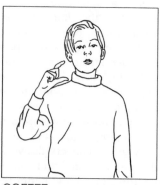

COFFEE

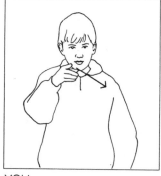

YOU

begins. The most common types of conversations are those where the conversational partner (C) asks about known things and gives the individual (I) help in answering, by using WHAT , for example, or giving a prompt, i.e. help or encouragement.

I: (Using signs) COFFEE
C: (Using signs and speech) YOU COFFEE (*You can have coffee*)

C: WHAT (*What do you want to do?*)
I: OUT WALK
C: JACKET (*Put on your jacket*)

There is no simple answer as to how this pattern should be broken, except in situations that are strictly structured or rit-ualised. However, it may be useful to try to find amusing and interesting topics. Situations that children and adults belong-ing to the alternative language group may find suitable to talk about are circumstances that the individual and conver-sational partner have experienced together, or perhaps com-mon friends. Using a photograph album and pictures taken in familiar situations is often a good way of beginning a longer conversation.

There is, as may be expected, a relationship between conversational skills and other linguistic skills. However, there are no fixed rules as to how many signs or spoken words the individual must master before attempts are made at conversing. Normally developed children in the early stages of language development, with very limited vocabu-laries, take part in simple dialogues with their parents and other adults. There has been some success in teaching autistic and severely mentally handicapped people, who had learned 40–80 signs which they seldom used sponta-neously, to participate in conversations.

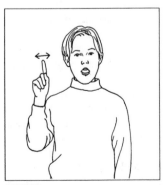

WHAT

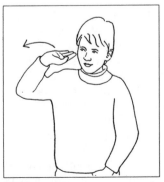

OUT

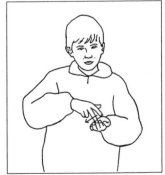

WALK

Routines, plans and scripts

In sign teaching, structuring and fixed routines are used to teach individuals what is going to happen. The structure helps the individuals to get an idea about what is happening, facilitates their understanding and use of the signs they are going to learn, and builds up their expectations. In general, people always have a set of expectations as to what different situations will contain, and what will happen. Descriptions of these situations are called *plans* or *scripts* (Schank and Abelson, 1977). Plans are more detailed than scripts. Plans contain a description of a specific course of events, while scripts describe a more general situation with possibilities for variation. In a communicative situation with strict structuring the description will be a plan, while a more flexible structure may be called a script.

Scripts have been used to describe the development of early dialogue skills among children who develop language normally, and strategies for developing conversational skills among individuals who belong to the alternative language group have for a large part been based on scripts. In reality this is a continuation of structuring and emphasising of routines. This means that the teacher both builds up a plan or a script and utilises it to make conversations.

The first conversations children normally take part in come about because adults structure and design conversations by prompting and coaxing answers out of the child. It is the adult (A) who *links* the child's (C) utterances together and produces a meaningful entity.

> A: *Yesterday you went to...*
> C:
> A: *You went to Grand...*
> C: *To Grandmother's*
> A: *And you travelled by...*
> C: *Train*

Typical conversations concern things one is in the process of doing, or has done. They may be about the food the adult is cooking, a visit, the children at nursery school, etc. Many conversations recur often, so that the child gradually learns what to say to the various cues. Some conversations are repeated on a daily basis.

Attempts should be made to establish similar conversations with people who have communication disorders. The conversational partner controls the course of the conversation and prompts for the individual's conversational turns, i.e. gives encouragement and helps the individual to answer. For some individuals who belong to the alternative language group, this may be a procedure they will require for the rest of their lives. For these individuals the greatest gain is to learn the role of conversational partner, and those in contact with them can gradually weave new elements into the conversation, elements that may lead to new learning.

Sommer, Whitman and Keogh (1988) taught six mentally handicapped and autistic young people to have a conversation about a game of quoits. They were between the ages of 8 and 25 and had little or no speech. Their sign vocabulary varied between 40 and 80 signs, but these signs were rarely used spontaneously. Seven signs were used in the teaching situation: YOU, I, WANT, (TO) PLAY, (TO) THROW, MORE and YES. The dialogue itself was formulated as a plan.

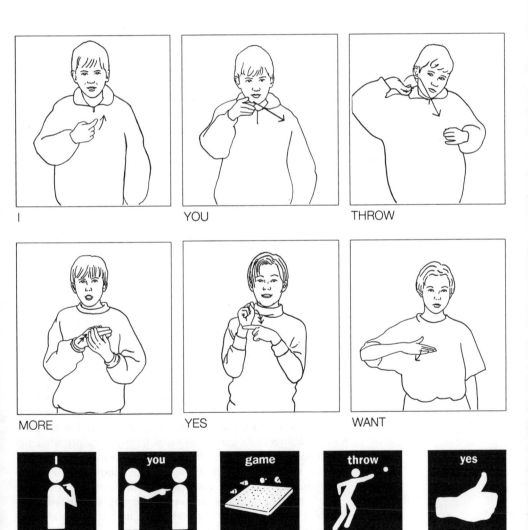

I   YOU   THROW

MORE   YES   WANT

I   you   game   throw   yes

P1: YOU WANT (TO) PLAY
P2: I WANT (TO) PLAY
P1: THROW
P2: (Throws)
P2: YOU THROW
P1: (Throws)
P1: YOU THROW
P2: (Throws)
P2: YOU THROW
P1: (Throws)
P2: PLAY MORE
P1: YES

To begin with, the conversation was performed with each of the young people and a teacher. Then the teacher helped the young people to perform the conversation together in pairs. The help they were given consisted of prompts if one of the participants stopped. Two of them learned to perform the whole sequence, while the remaining four learned to perform parts of it. The quoit dialogue was based on a situation in which the individuals generally interacted, and where the sign sentences fulfilled a functional role. They continued to use some of the signs when they played quoits, even after the training sessions ended.

The two most capable individuals in this study had previously taken part in a study where, in a similar manner, they had to learn to perform a conversation about orange juice and biscuits. They learned to use a number of the sign sentences together with the teacher but not with one another (Keogh et al., 1987). In this study they used 15 signs and three different plans, and there is reason to believe that this was too complex. At the same time it is conceivable that the good results achieved by the two individuals in the second study was due to their previous experience.

In both studies a plan was used, i.e. a dialogue written beforehand, rather than a script. The aim in such situations should be to gradually change the dialogue to a script with greater flexibility. There is reason to believe that this will lead to increased generalisation and more spontaneous use than was the case in these studies. The strategy of teaching conversational skills with the aid of a plan is, however, totally new, and the approach needs to be tested in a variety of situations before one can say with any certainty what significance this method may have for developing conversational skills in everyday settings. In the study carried out by Sommer et al. (1988) only parts of the conversation were used more generally. In particular the comment YOU THROW was omitted, probably because this remark was redundant since the turn of the next player was signalled by

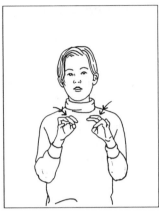

FINISHED

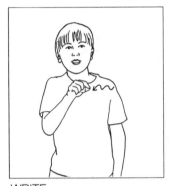

WRITE

the fact that the first player had finished throwing. Perhaps it would have been better to introduce the sign FINISHED into the conversation. It is also conceivable that the participants would like to make a note of the number of quoits that had landed on the peg. Thus, WRITE and FINISHED could have been introduced at the appropriate stages of the game.

The little experience there is in terms of the usefulness of direct training of conversational skills is mixed. However, there is reason to try this approach with individuals who have learned a number of signs. In institutions for mentally handicapped people almost all communication is between the residents and staff members. A significant argument for trying out conversational training is that its aim is to get individuals with impaired communication skills to communicate with one other.

Supportive language group

Conversational skills have not been a chief concern in the teaching of individuals who belong to the supportive language group either, even though it is expected that they will begin to take part in conversations.

For children who belong to the supportive language group, first conversations are often a frustrating experience. This applies in particular to children with developmental language disorders and other individuals who have such extensive articulatory problems that it is difficult for the listener to understand what is being said. Conversations tend to come to a standstill. These individuals will generally answer yes to questions, even though they have not understood what it is they are being asked.

Even for adults in close contact with these children, their speech is inadequate for them to be understood: the adults depend on situational clues in order to comprehend what the children are trying to say. In situations where there are no such clues, very little will be understood. For example, parents relate that it is especially difficult to understand their children when they are out driving (Schjølberg, 1984). The problems adults encounter when trying to understand these children will often lead to their answering yes and no to questions – in the same way as the children – in the hope that the reply they give will be the correct one. This way of answering does not encourage continued conversation, and the children will often stop communicating when they experience that they receive incorrect and meaningless answers. The adults, in an effort to keep the conversation going when they have not understood what the children are saying, take control of the conversation by asking the children questions, or by deciding for themselves the course of events. This exerts pressure on

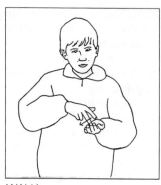

WALK

the children's communicative ability, in order for them to be able to do what they want. If it is the case that the adults always decide, the children may find that the time spent with them is uninteresting.

The objective of the teaching is to make it easier for the children to participate in conversations, and for them to experience that others understand them. Using graphic or manual signs helps the conversational partner understand, so that the conversation does not come to a halt so easily and is not diverted from its objective by the adults' attempts to understand what the children meant. This may provide the children with increased opportunities for indirect learning and give them greater benefit from contact with adults.

The teaching does not differ appreciably from that given to the alternative language group, although strategies employed with the expressive language group may also be utilised (see below). Emphasis should be given to dialogues in natural settings, in the form of structured conversations about a clearly defined topic. The conversations will then begin by establishing a topic, for example by saying: *Let's talk about your bicycle* or: *You know that walk we're going on tomorrow?* To make sure that the topic has been understood, and that the children are attentive, one should make sure that they confirm the topic. This may be clear if the children say BICYCLE or WALK. To make it easier for the adults to understand, scripts may be useful. This means that *new* situations are designed that are easy to grasp and understand but where the children are able to make a contribution, i.e. say something that the person with whom they are communicating does not know.

As well as using signs and establishing a topic of conversation, the intelligibility of the speech of children with articulatory disorders may be improved by designing situations in which the adults have several situational cues for what a child is interested in. Such situations may be arranged simply: e.g. a child and the adult play together with the same toys from day to day but the game differs somewhat. The adult is encouraged to comment on what the child does with the toys. In such a situation the child will experience that more of what he or she says is understood, without having to resort to boring repetition, and the adult will gradually learn more about how the child speaks and articulates sounds. Conversations where pictures or other forms of help will provide the conversation with a framework, and the child contributes with information that is unknown to the conversational partner, are also suitable.

It is essential that the partners in the conversation change roles. The teacher or the adult should not always be the one to ask questions while the speech-impaired child answers. The child should also ask for information, encourage activity, etc. Since the conversation has a tendency to come to a standstill, the child will generally have little experience of keeping to one topic of conversation. One important aim is therefore to help the child to keep to one topic and follow it up in the conversation. Role-play may be useful. However, the play situation may easily become stereotypical and ritualised if the adult makes the same comments each time. By changing roles, the adult's chaining, which is so important to keep the conversation going, will gradually be broken down. A larger share of the communicative responsibility may be transferred to the child in a positive manner.

Since the children in the supportive language group are difficult to understand, people around them often assume that they do not have anything of significance to say. Part of the teaching is therefore to demonstrate to the people in contact with the children that they are able to participate in conversations and do have something to say. This helps to lay the basis for a more natural form of language learning, which for this group usually will replace the formalised teaching over time.

For some children who belong to the supportive language group, for example children with Down's syndrome, the problem of establishing conversations in which the children take an equal share of the communicative initiative is related to the fact that the children need a long time to react to what other people are doing and what is otherwise happening in the situation. The problem the adults will experience is having to wait long enough so that the children have a chance to take their turn. The best way of remedying this is to encourage the conversational partners to wait a little longer than usual, and let them be convinced by personal experience that this kind of waiting is not in vain. To ensure that the experiences will be positive, the waiting may take place in established situations where it is highly likely that the children will take the initiative to communicate.

Expressive language group

There are a number of circumstances that combine to produce problems for children and adults who belong to the expressive language group when participating in meaningful conversation. Above all, the different communication aids have practical consequences which, together with the user's motor impairment, produce physical restrictions in terms of how the conversations may be kept going. The type of aid that is used may have great significance for the course of conversation. However, poor conversational skills are also the result of a inadequate teaching and unfortunate experiences individual have had when communicating with others. Conversational partners often act in such a way that conversations become more difficult and have little meaning. They pretend to understand utterances although in fact they have not, they answer questions aimed at individuals instead of allowing them to answer for themselves, and they tend to raise their voices when speaking to them (Shane and Cohen, 1981; Kraat, 1985). Similar strategies are found when speaking to people who have a different native language (Ferguson and Debose, 1977).

Some of the most important problems that must be overcome are the individuals' lack of communicative initiative, passive communicative style, slow communication and inadequate communicative strategies. In reality these are intertwined. A good solution requires as a rule that both individuals and conversational partners learn to act in new ways, that considerable thought is given when choosing a communication aid, and that circumstances are practically designed so that the aid can be used as effectively as possible.

For members of the expressive language group who have a good understanding of language, the development of conversational skills is the most important aim of teaching. It is usually not the lack of linguistic skills that places restrictions on users of communication aids, but rather the lack of opportunities to use what they know. They do not need language teaching in the traditional sense, instead they need training in the technical and functional use of the aid. Traditional language intervention of a kind they do not need may lead to passivity and dependence. Their experience with communication has played a significant role in the development of a passive communicative style. The significance of learning good strategies in order to initiate and maintain conversations seems to have been underestimated. It was assumed that functional and varied use of communication aids would follow once the sign system and the aid had been mastered technically (Harris, 1982; Kraat, 1985). An emphasis on conversational strategies may help increase awareness of this problem, and thereby lead to less learned dependency.

Individuals who belong to the expressive language group are often physically disabled and have difficulty in performing a large number of commonplace activities that require motor skills. They often have best control over language, and linguistic comments replace a number of activities that occur naturally in ordinary interaction, for example pointing, showing and manipulating objects. The development of conversational skills is therefore of vital importance if this group is to be able to participate in a range of social contexts.

The teaching employed to develop better conversational skills may be divided into *environmental strategies, partner strategies* and *conversational strategies*. Environmental strategies and partner strategies aim at increasing the individual's participation in conversational situations, reducing routine situations and ensuring that conversational partners adapt to the language-impaired individuals. Conversational strategies are strategies that the individuals themselves may use to make their communication more effective.

Environmental strategies

Many motor-impaired individuals have greater mastery of language skills than of motor skills. They should therefore by rights participate in more communicative situations than others. In reality, however, they participate in fewer such situations. The conversations they have are often with professional helpers, and a large number of the communicative situations in which they participate are routine situations. This is partly because physically disabled individuals spend longer periods of time on routine activities than other people, but is also due to the fact that parents of speech-impaired children prefer to communicate in such situations because it is in these settings that they understand their children best (Culp, 1982).

Routine situations hinder participation in new situations. One way of making the most of the environment is to find new situations where conversation may take place or form part of the activity. The situations can if necessary be made easier for the ordinary conversational partners to follow, so that they experience success in the communicative situation. At the same time it is important that the situation is not designed in such a way that too few demands are made on the aided speaker. For example, parents of disabled children use their knowledge about the children in order to guess what it is they want. The children take part in few activities, and the parents are familiar with most of them. It is easy for the parents to guess the children's wishes, and the content of such conversations can quickly become repetitive and monotonous. Not everything in the situation should be predictable. The conversational partners should have a need to know what the individuals are communicating, so that they have a communicative responsibility. Lack of communicative responsibility and genuine communication are common barriers to the development of conversational skills (Glennen and Calculator, 1985).

It is common practice to use an information booklet that is carried between home and nursery school or school. An information booklet can be useful in many situations, and is often used with individuals who belong to the supportive and alternative language groups. It ensures that important information is systematically conveyed between home and school. However, it can also rob the individuals of communicative responsibility, because, for example, they will be unable to choose what is related from home or school. Only those topics mentioned in the book will be discussed. Many of the questions asked of the individuals will not be genuine, since the conversational partners will know or can make a good guess at what the answer will be. In this way the individuals will have few clues to tell them whether they are communicating well or poorly. Communicative setbacks may also lead to positive learning, but this assumes that the individuals know what was wrong and what can be changed in order to make the communication more effective.

An increase in the number of different communicative situations implies an opening up of society for disabled individuals. Communication should occur not only at home, at nursery school, school, work and in other familiar situations, but also with unknown people, on the street, in cafes, shops, meeting places, cinemas, etc. However, it is not always just a case of throwing individuals into new situations. They are often apprehensive about being exposed to people who are not used to individuals who use communication aids, and may be fearful and reject new situations. It may therefore be necessary to begin by giving the individuals a good overview of the situation and what is likely to happen there, so that they can feel more secure. Role-playing may be one way of preparing for new situations.

> Becky is a 9-year-old girl with cerebral palsy. She has some speech but it is almost unintelligible. She uses a communication book with 200 Rebus signs. The book contains mini communication boards with different domains (art, snacks, assembly, etc.). She often goes to Burger King with her parents but has never ordered anything there herself. First she talks with her teacher about what happens at Burger King. One must wait to be served, order exactly what one wants, and pay. Becky and her teacher then make a domain board for Burger King. In the classroom they make a model of Burger King, where a school-mate plays the role of waiter. When the 'waiter' asks what she wants, she points at the adapted communication board in her book. She practises telling the waiter whether he has understood her correctly or not. When she goes to Burger King with her friend who played the role of waiter, she gets the hamburger she wants, without any difficulties (Mills and Higgins, 1984).

> Martin is a 12-year-old boy with cerebral palsy. He has several communication books with limited vocabularies and also uses an electronic writing instrument where what he writes is printed on paper. However, the writing process is extremely slow. Martin

likes to read but has never been to the library. First he and his teacher talk about what it is like at the library, and they discuss the process of borrowing books. He practises writing a few sentences he will find useful, such as 'Where are the books about lions?' and 'How many books can I borrow?' Then a friend from his class plays the role of librarian. He asks questions and Martin answers. The following day they go to the library, where Martin easily masters the new situation (Higgins and Mills, 1986).

It is important to stress that role-playing should not be a replacement for real situations; it is precisely pretend situations that characterise many of the experiences of disabled individuals who use aided communication. The role-playing is only intended as a means of making it easier for an individual to begin to take part in the real situation. This objective of the role-playing should be clear from the outset, for both teacher and learner.

Generally speaking, aided speakers participate less in conversations than others. For children and adolescents, the vast majority of their conversations are with adults (Harris, 1982). Interaction and communication with peers should therefore be increased. Situations where children interact with adults differ from situations in which children interact with one another. Children and adolescents who use communication aids also seem to have more varied conversations with their peers than with adults (Sutton, 1982). Conversations with peers also give the individuals access to a youth culture. Particular care should be taken to design activities that may take place without the help of an adult, for example role-playing and games. The adult should refrain from interrupting unnecessarily, even if conflicts and arguments arise. Just like other people, users of communication aids should also experience such situations and learn how to deal with them. Shielding disabled children more than others against such circumstances means that they do not have the opportunity to gain commonplace experiences and learn to tackle everyday situations. For adolescents, school-friends or other peers may be responsible for helping the individuals and including them in leisure-time activities. As far as possible, these should be activities that are popular among young people, encouraging the individuals to play as equal a role as possible despite the fact that they are motor impaired. Visits to the cinema, sports events, homework, visits to cafés, listening to records and hanging around on street corners are examples of such activities.

Telecommunication

More communication does not necessarily mean that the communication *must* be face-to-face. For motor-impaired people who have difficulty in moving, telecommunication is an important opportunity to participate in conversation. Conversations may take place directly, i.e. with a text telephone or computer, and with script or synthetic speech. It is also possible to communicate with graphic signs (Tronconi, 1989). However, modern computer technology also provides opportunities for other types of 'conversation'; conversations in the form of computer conferences or bulletin boards.

A computer conference consists of a computer linked to the telecommunication network. The participants use their own computers hooked up to a modem to communicate with the host computer. Thus, those participating in the conference or 'conversation' need not be in the same location. Nor do all the participants need to be present at the same time, but because new comments build on previous ones, the computer conference resembles a group conversation. The participants can see what the others have written, and write their own comments when it suits them.

The advantage of computer conferences for people who use communication aids is that they need not communicate quickly. They can write what they want at their own speed, and are not dependent on others to interpret for them. However, they must be able to use orthographic script (Magnusson and Lundman, 1987).

Partner strategies

In addition to their own role, partners in conversation with communication aid users must often take an active part in formulating what the individuals want to say. The partners interpret elements as they are indicated by the aided speakers, assemble these elements, and to some extent, guess at what the individuals are saying before they have finished forming the sentence. The conversational partners are therefore the active participants, whether they are speaking or listening. The conversational partners' strategies and degree of competence will vary. Since the conversational partners have a double role, training them is an important means of providing communication aid users with better conversational skills.

In a typical conversation between an aided and a natural speaker it is the natural speaker who takes the initiative to change subjects and control the conversation. This is done in a way that may best be described as a *simplification strategy*, i.e. the conversational partner limits the topic of conversation and what the aided speaker may say. This may make it easy for an aided speaker to be part of the conversation, but difficult for him or her to make a contribution. In many instances one gets the impression that the helping role of the conversational partner deludes him or her into underestimating the aided speaker. Particularly among conversational partners who are not aware of their special role, one may find that they talk down to aided speakers and do not take into account what the individuals actually know and understand (Blau, 1983; Shane and Cohen, 1981).

The aided speakers' contribution to the conversation consists for the most part of giving replies, and the conversational partners restrict the number of possible answers through the way they pose the questions. In spite of the fact that the communication takes time, the contributions made by the speech-impaired individuals are limited. It is the conversational partners who take the initiative and choose the topic of conversation. Sutton (1982) found that the speaker took the initiative 84 per cent of the time, while 10–27-year-old users of Blissymbols took the initiative to communicate only 16 per cent of the time. Similarly, Light (1985) found that the mothers of 3–6-year-old Blissymbol users took the initiative 85 per cent of the time.

Time to say something

A conversation always takes much longer if communication aids are used than if both participants are able to speak naturally. If the conversation has several turns and contains a mutual exchange of information and opinions, the time taken will increase considerably. If the individuals wish to say something that is outside the bounds of ordinary routines, it may take them a long time to express themselves. The length of time this takes leads to problems in saying things that are important. This is the main reason for the asymmetrical conversational structure and the strategies generally used by conversational partners. Many conversational partners find it difficult to wait. Light (1985) found that mothers of 3–6-year-old children began to speak after 1–2 seconds. Pauses of more than 1 second were followed by speech from the mothers 92.5 per cent of the time. The children, who needed longer to be able to speak with the help of their Blissboards, only had time to answer yes–no questions (see below), which they were able to answer quickly by vocalising, nodding or shaking their heads. The importance of giving the individuals sufficient time was well demonstrated by the fact that the mother of the child who communicated the most also waited the longest, as much as 47 seconds. While the average number of communicative initiatives on the part of the children in the course of 20 minutes was 11, this particular child had 45 initiatives. Similarly, Glennen and Calculator (1985) found an increase in communicative initiative for two children aged 9 and 12 once the conversational partners had been taught to wait.

In order to give users of aided communication an opportunity to control the course of conversation better, and contribute to the conversation on a more equal footing, it is first and foremost important that they be given the time they need to say what they want to say. This implies that the conversational partners must wait long enough before they begin to interpret or guess at what the individuals are saying, or take the communicative initiative, be it a continuation of the conversation or a change of topic.

Guessing

In order to speed up the conversation, it is usual for conversational partners to guess a word before it is fully spelled out, or whole sentences before all the signs are produced or pointed at. Most utterances made by children who use communication aids and graphic signs are single sign utterances (Sutton 1982; Harris, 1982). This is partly due to the fact that a large part of the children's utterances are replies to questions, but is also due to the fact that conversational partners guess after the first sign. The listeners guess what the individuals wish to say, and express this for them. Guessing in this way may be a good strategy for making conversations more effective, but it may also lead to individuals being unable to express themselves. The interpretation of words and sentences generally takes place one element at a time, which means that listeners may have to remember the letters in the word that is being spelled out and the words or signs that have already been articulated. This can be quite difficult, especially if a conversational partner has to spend some time figuring out a sign analogy or spelling out a long word. The utterances need not be especially long before mistakes are made. If a conversational partner guesses wrongly, and is too preoccupied and inattentive to realise it, the result can be both frustrating and humiliating.

B: *When's the holiday?*
A: (Points at the communication board containing Blissymbols) *MONTH O.*
B: *MONTH O? I don't get you, Joey.*
B: *Try to form a sentence with it.*
A: (Pounds three times on the letter) *O. O. O.*
B: *Does the month begin with an O?*
A: *Yes.*
B: *October?*
A: *Yes?*
B: *So. A holiday in October. Uh, let's see. Oh, I know. Thanksgiving* (Canadian). *Do you like turkey as much as I do?*
A: (Points at the board) *H.*
B: *H? I don't understand. What does H have to do with Thanksgiving?*

A: (Does not answer)
B: *Do you know why we celebrate Thanksgiving? About the Pilgrims and Plymouth Rock and all of that?*
A: (Expresses frustration)

In this example the listener guessed that the user meant Thanksgiving, while the user was actually thinking about Halloween. B showed no interest in A's attempts to rectify the misunderstanding, but merely continued on his own track (Silverman, Kates and McNaughton, 1978). B's patronising attitude is emphasised by the fact that Thanksgiving is well known in North America, and something learned at an early stage at school. The major problem was that the conversational partner had not taken care to get confirmation that he had guessed correctly. Such confirmation should be an essential part of a conversational partner's strategy and will guarantee that misunderstandings are not built on in the conversation.

In some instances guessing may lead to dependency and hinder development of good conversational strategies.

> Larry is 26 years old and has cerebral palsy. He can speak, but his speech is difficult to understand. In order to make himself understood to people who have difficulty comprehending what he says, he uses a letter board. He spoke with a Swedish girl who did not know him, and who did not understand that he said the word hospital although this word is very similar in Norwegian and Swedish. Larry began to spell out the word but gave up after h-o-s-p-i. Since his conversational partner had not guessed the word, Larry began to spell the word from the beginning instead of spelling out the whole word. This caused great problems in the communicative situation and meant that it took him a long time to finish telling the joke he had started.

This discussion is not meant as an argument against employing guessing as a strategy. Many users of communication aids prefer their conversational partner to guess what they are trying to say before they have finished formulating the utterance. It can be a good strategy on the part of the conversational partner to guess what is being said before the utterance is fully articulated, and people who know the user well are best able do this effectively. When graphic signs are used, this kind of guessing is natural since the conversational partner usually interprets what the user is saying with the aid of the signs. Even though guessing is often expedient, it is essential to make sure that it is confirmed. It is also important that individuals are able to master other strategies so that the guessing does not cause them to become dependent on their conversational partner, and they learn to express themselves on occasions when conversational partners fail to guess or the guessing leads them nowhere.

Yes–no questions

It is typical in conversations between aided and natural speakers that the users of communication aids have a responsive role, i.e. they answer questions and requests from their conversational partner. In a study carried out by Sutton (1982), questions accounted for 34 per cent and 2 per cent of the conversational partners' and the children's utterances, respectively. In a study of adult communication aid users Wexler, Blau, Leslie and Dore (1983) found that the aided speakers produced eight requests and questions and 163 answers, while the conversational partners had 285 questions and challenges and eight answers.

A large part of the communication from natural to aided speakers consists of yes–no questions. Sutton (1982) found that 16 per cent of utterances from those who spoke to 10–27-year-old Blissymbol users were yes–no questions. In a study carried out by Culp (1982), 40 per cent of the utterances made by aided speakers were answers to yes–no questions. In addition, a large number of the questions posed by conversational partners are about circumstances to which they already know the answer (Light, 1985; Sutton, 1982). Often the aided speakers are aware of this, and the conversations have little meaning.

It is not uncommon for questions to be followed up by more specific sub-questions before the individuals have been given the chance to answer. In the following example the teacher (T) begins by asking a question that could have been a good starting point for a conversation, but ruins a possible conversation with the pupil (P) before it has even begun (Harris, 1982).

> T: *What did you do last night?*
> P: (Begins to formulate an answer on the communication board).
> T: *Did you go home?*
> T: *Did you go to the cinema?*
> T: *Did you watch television?*
> T: *Did you watch Walt Disney?*
> T: *Did your brother come?*

In order to increase the number of contributions to the conversation on the part of the individual, conversational partners should use fewer yes–no questions when it is not necessary to use these to find out what individuals mean, e.g. because they do not have the signs they need to be able to express what they want. As far as possible questions should be open, i.e. of the type 'what', 'who', 'where', etc., which will prompt more than just yes–no answers, but the general aim should be to reduce the number of questions.

Corrections

Many children and adolescents seldom use their communication aid spontaneously. To make them use the aid more often, professionals and parents may encourage the use of the aid in situations where the individuals have managed to make themselves understood in other ways (Harris, 1982).

> T: *What do you want?*
> P: (Points to the ball).
> T: *No, tell me with your board.*
> P: (Points to the ball again).
> T: *How can you tell me with your board.*
> P: (Puts head down on lap tray).

Functional teaching does consist of teaching individuals new ways to express themselves in situations where they are already capable of communicating effectively. The aim is for them to learn to communicate in situations where their mastery is insufficient. Forcing individuals to use a communication aid when this is not functional, in the belief that they will become better at communicating because they are pointing at a graphic sign instead of an object, has little purpose. The individual in the example above had mastered the use of the graphic sign, and the 'correction' was merely felt to be unnecessary and a form of nagging. Such situations produce negative experiences which may rob the individuals of their motivation to communicate.

Conversational strategies

Starting and ending conversations

In order to begin a conversation, individuals must have ways of attracting a conversational partner's attention. If they are able to vocalise, make clicking noises with the tongue, say some words, or have a communication aid that uses synthetic speech, this will generally be no problem. However, for individuals who are dependent on visual contact, it can be extremely difficult to attract the conversational partner's attention. Attempts at communication are often overlooked, especially on occasions when it is the individual who takes the initiative. To be successful, the potential conversational partner must be looking in the right direction. When the individual is responding to a question, however, the person who has asked the question will also direct his or her attention at the person who is going to answer.

Mothers of pre-school children who use Blissymbols take the initiative to communicate 85 per cent of the time

(Light, 1985). Conversational partners of adult communication users take the initiative to communicate 79 per cent of the time (Wexler et al., 1983). Calculator and Dollaghan (1982) found that 20–40 per cent of communicative initiatives on the part of motor-impaired individuals was overlooked in the classroom. One reason for this, among others, is that many people with extensive motor handicaps produce involuntary sounds or movements that people around them become used to and ignore. Many individuals who are able to articulate sounds have difficulty in doing so when it is important for them to express themselves. In order that individuals can be sure they will be able to attract a conversational partner's attention, it may be necessary for them to use a type of alarm system. A form of buzzer or bell can be practical, but a small speech machine that says: *Hello,* or something similar, is better. For people who use communication aids that employ synthetic speech, ready-made opening phrases may make it easy to begin a conversation, e.g.: *Hi, I'd like to talk to you.* Touching may also be a way of attracting someone's attention, but for people who do not know the individual, this may seem threatening (Yoder and Kraat, 1983).

It is not uncommon for a communication aid user always to use the same topic as a means of initiating a conversation (Shane, Lipshultz and Shane, 1982). This leads to dull conversations, and the conversational partner becomes bored. In such cases it will be useful to teach individuals to use different subjects to begin conversations.

Since the conversation is to a great extent dominated by the conversational partner, he or she also generally decides when the conversation will end. This may happen either sooner or later than the individual would wish. It is not always easy for individuals to withdraw from a situation, or demonstrate in one way or another that they wish to stop. It is therefore essential that they are given strategies that they can utilise when they wish to end a conversation, for example, by teaching them to say END CONVERSATION or some such phrase. If they want to say more, they must also know how to signal this. It can easily be done by saying SPEAK MORE or NO END. Even though the individuals use graphic signs, it is likely that they will have suitable signs on their board; if not, it should be no problem to provide them with the necessary signs. However, it is not very likely that they themselves have much experience of ending conversations, so they must be taught how they can use the signs to do so.

Breakdowns and repairs

A large share of the utterances produced in aided communication are misunderstood and lead to a breakdown in

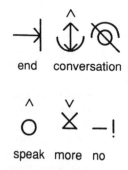

end   conversation

speak more no

talk/speak

communication. The breakdowns are often due to the fact that the amount of time individuals spend expressing themselves make the listener lose concentration and thereby lose track of what is being said, but imprecise pointing and faults on the part of the user may also cause misunderstandings. To make sure that these breakdowns do not lead to the whole conversation breaking down, it is essential that individuals have strategies he can use to signal that a misunderstanding has occurred and remedy this. Breakdowns in communication may also be due to problems encountered by individuals when attempting to express themselves with a limited number of signs or words.

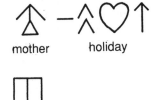

mother   holiday

book

> A 12-year-old girl with cerebral palsy was going home for her Christmas holidays and said with the aid of Blissymbols, MOTHER HOLIDAY BOOK. She refused to leave the school and continued to repeat the same three signs. After an hour her teacher discovered that the girl wanted to take home the 'report card' that he had read aloud for her, where it said that she had made great progress.

It is not uncommon for people with limited means of expressing themselves to allow a misunderstanding to pass because they do not know how to repair or remedy it, or because it would take too long to rectify (Yoder and Kraat, 1983). Children between the ages of 3 and 6 have few repair strategies (Light, 1985). In the above example it was the girl's persistence that led to her finally taking her report card home with her. However, she was unable to rephrase what she wanted to say, and it is unlikely that she had received sufficient teaching in how to clarify situations that were not understood.

The most common strategy used when repairing misunderstandings is to point at the same sign once more or spell the word again. This is a good strategy to use if the listener did not see which sign the aided speaker used, or lost track of the spelling the first time. Another strategy is to reformulate what was said. This is especially important when using signs, where it is often necessary for individuals to paraphrase in order to express what they want to say. It is important that children are taught to use repair strategies, and also receive teaching in how they can make conversational partners aware that they have misconstrued or misunderstood what was said. Repetition might be construed as the next word or utterance, and conversational partners might be uncertain about where the misunderstanding lies. There should therefore be a sign for 'misunderstanding' on the board, which clearly says that the interpretation or perception of what has been said is incorrect. In synthetic speech an utterance such as: *That wasn't exactly what I*

wrong

meant might be used. Individuals should learn to use this sign before they begin to repeat signs or words, or try to clarify or paraphrase what they intended to say.

Taking turns

To contribute to maintaining a conversation, individuals must be able to take their turn in the conversation. Users of communication aids often lose their turn because they take so long getting started that their conversational partners do not take the time to wait. In a study by Light (1985) the mothers used almost all the opportunities they had to take their turn, while the children used only half of their chances. Most of the opportunities the children used were when they answered questions. There are also obligatory turns in a conversation, where the conversational partner prompts the other to say something, e.g. to answer a question. Aided speakers do not even always take these obligatory turns (Calculator and Luchko, 1983).

Part of the reason that users of communication aids do not enter the conversation is that the switching of turns is often signalled by non-verbal signals, which they do not master. These may take the form of intonation and facial expression. Among motor-impaired individuals, such signals are often misunderstood. An attempt at pointing may be regarded as a warding off. If the individual is unable to hold his or her head up, this may be perceived as an indication of a lack of interest and the conversation will be ended (Morris, 1981; Yoder and Kraat, 1983).

In addition, there is the imbalance in how much is said by each of the conversational partners. The conversational partner may have long exchanges, while the aided speakers will generally only have one exchange for each turn they take (Light, 1985). This will result in the children and adults in the expressive language group experiencing problems in conversing in an everyday, ordinary way. Conversing, making small comments while the conversational partner is speaking, and telling funny stories and cracking jokes are some of the most difficult things to do for an individual who depends on a communication board and a helper. The chances individuals have of expressing more than they generally say every day in the same situations depends on there being plenty of time, and on their conversational partners being attentive and careful not to decide too much of the content of the conversation.

Topic–comment

One possible way of improving conversations is if individuals and their conversational partners learn to use a

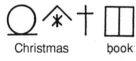

Christmas   book

topic–comment structure in the conversation. This means that the individual and the conversational partner first decide upon the topic of conversation, and that what is said later in the utterance or conversation is in the form of a comment on or a specification of the topic. Such a construction makes it easier for the conversational partner to understand, and reduces the likelihood of misunderstanding. When it takes time to construct the sentence, for example CHRISTMAS BOOK, CHRISTMAS will bring to the conversational partner's attention that the individual wishes to say something about that season. Thus the next sign will lead the conversational partner to understand that the individual was given a book as a Christmas present. A topic–comment strategy will increase the likelihood that the person who interprets or guesses what is being said will guess correctly.

The topic–comment structure is typical of the language used by people who have different native languages and therefore have difficulty in communicating with one another. If they communicate regularly with one another, they will develop a common language. These languages, which are generally used in trading areas, are called pidgin languages (Broch and Jahr, 1981). Since a topic–comment structure is used in situations where people have difficulty in communicating, there is reason to believe that this strategy is also well suited to people who use communication aids. It represents both a strategy for initiating a conversation or introducing a new subject and a means of gaining control over the content of the conversation. At the same time it is an economical strategy, enabling the use of fewer words, which also makes the strategy useful.

The teaching of individuals who use communication aids has often been characterised by a normative attitude which requires the 'correct' use of language. The use of topic–comment construction of sentences and conversations differs from common notions of how language should be. In order to use a topic–comment structure, it is necessary to break consciously with the normative conception of 'correct' speech. This may be necessary in order to ensure individuals who use communication aids the most effective possible communication in as many situations and settings as possible. In conversations with people who are unfamiliar with communication aids, it may nonetheless be necessary for the user of a communication aid to adapt linguistically. This is generally done by using a more elaborate or 'correct' language (Morningstar, 1981).

Chapter 11
The language
environment

Individuals who learn augmentative communication spend little time in a teaching situation compared to the time they spend in their natural environment. If the teaching is to have any purpose, it must help the individual to be able to use and develop communication skills in everyday situations. A lack of knowledge about the system, and insensitive communicative strategies on the part of conversational partners, however, means that many augmentative communication users become *communicative under-achievers*. They are often not credited with an ability to communicate, or with having anything to communicate about. This means that the people in the individuals' environment must learn how they communicate, and be given the opportunity to communicate with them to find out what they are capable of.

Children who learn to speak normally do so through interaction with a supportive language environment. An ordinary language environment consists of family members, staff members at the nursery school, and other adults and children in the child's immediate surroundings. Individuals who are taught augmentative communication have also grown up in normal language environments, but they have been unable to acquire language within the ordinary framework. It is therefore necessary to adapt the environment specially for them. The adaptation should include as many of the people in close contact with the child as possible, and thus entails teaching the family and nursery school, school or institution staff, as well as other significant people in touch with the child.

Adapting the environment

One of the aims of an adapted environment is to get the people in contact with individuals to react to a greater part of their behaviour as though it were communicative. On the whole, one is particularly aware of the sounds individuals make, though it is easier to overlook communicative efforts where individuals use, for example, arm movements or posture. An adapted environment may make it easier to over-interpret individuals' movements, facial expressions and posture. This increases the likelihood that the individual will be reacted to, which in turn fosters self-initiated activity.

For infants and young disabled children, the intervention is usually aimed at encouraging interaction and communication. The interventionary measures are directed at how the parents and others react to the child. Augmentative communication teaching does not generally begin during the first year of life. The use of graphic and manual signs is generally discussed only if the parents broach the subject, and is then considered a possibility only if the child does not begin to speak normally.

On occasions where it is certain that a child is *at risk* of developing inadequate speech, discussion about using augmentative communication may begin when the child is only a few months old. The use of manual signs requires some teaching, and it is an advantage if key people in the environment have learned some signs before the child is expected to begin using them. It may also be useful to prepare older children in the nursery school the child attends, or will soon attend, by teaching them a number of signs. From very early on parents and other adults may help by performing manual signs when the child shows interest in objects and activities in the environment.

Graphic signs can also be introduced in the same gradual way, so that the signs become a part of the language environment before the child is expected to use them. In this way the environment will become familiar along with the signs, and the child will experience less pressure from expectations when they are introduced.

The consequences of environmental adaptation for older children, adolescents and adults will depend on their linguistic abilities. For people with little language comprehension and a poor ability to express themselves, over-interpretation will still play an important role. For individuals with better language skills, it is most important to ensure that they are able to converse with people who understand them. This may, for example, be done by teaching potential communication partners, through planned 'incidental learning' and by making people in the environment realise what the individuals are capable of.

Individuals with extensive motor impairment often have such fixed routines that they have few opportunities to communicate. The objective for these individuals is to create a more varied everyday situation and produce communicative situations in which the conversational partners do not always know in advance what will be said.

The use of speech

One should always speak while performing manual or graphic signs, so that the sign learner has the opportunity to relate the sign to the spoken word. Using speech and signs has improved language comprehension for a number of individuals. For other individuals the accompanying speech seems to have neither a positive nor negative effect (Clark, Remmington and Light, 1986). Thus the conclusion in terms of whether speech should be used seems quite clear: it is always correct to use speech in association with signs.

Simple or complex language

The question of simple or complex language is one of whether the person communicating with a language-impaired individual should use simplified speech, or speak normally.

Shortened sentences do not appear to lead to improved comprehension on the part of mentally handicapped individuals who themselves generally produce one-word utterances. Experimental studies of children with normal language development have produced mixed results. In one study in which children with an average utterance length of under two words were supposed to follow more or less linguistically well-formulated instructions, Petretic and Tweeneny (1977) found that the normal well-formulated sentences would more likely lead to the correct action. Shortening sentences and omitting function words did not lead to improved comprehension. In a similar study Shipley, Gleitman and Smith (1969) found that children who themselves chiefly used one-word utterances reacted more frequently to shortened and simplified utterances than to utterances that were well formulated.

Because it is unnatural to speak in 'telegraphese', it seems best to use complete but simple sentences. The comprehension and use of passive sentences and utterances containing long subordinate clauses appear at a late stage in normal development, and are probably so difficult that it is best to avoid using them. It is essential for speech to be natural, so that adults feel comfortable and can direct their attention to the individual instead of being preoccupied with speaking correctly.

It is common for the signs to serve as a support for the speech rather than being used to express whole sentences.

When manual signs are used, small words and function words are generally omitted. This makes it easier to use manual signs, but individuals who learn augmentative communication should also be given the opportunity to learn prepositions and other function words once they have reached the appropriate linguistic level.

The way the conversational partner speaks determines which role the individual will play in the conversation. Even physically disabled individuals with good language comprehension and a communication board with a reasonable number of signs receive a disproportionate number of yes—no questions (Sutton, 1982; Basil, 1986). To provide individuals with an opportunity to use a greater number of signs and a more varied language, the people with whom they are in contact must be aware of the way they themselves use language. This means that they should vary their language, and, for example, increase the number of comments they make and ask open questions when speaking with aided speakers.

Models

A good language environment consists of people who use the expressive form the learner uses and who act as language models. It is natural to use signs as a means of support when speaking to individuals who are learning manual signs. However, people do not usually use a board as a means of helping individuals to comprehend speech when they converse with communication board users (Bruno and Bryen, 1986).

It is not uncommon for other children in the school or nursery school to learn some manual signs. They generally use these to tell sign users that they are going to eat, go for a walk, etc. Graphic signs may be used in the same way as manual signs, and some training is also necessary here. Although a number of graphic sign systems, e.g. PIC signs, seem easy to understand, it is still possible for children to misunderstand them. The fact that the signs are something the children have to learn, and that they are not merely incidental pictures, makes them more interesting for the other children. In this way the status of the sign system is enhanced, as is that of the child who uses it.

When people in the individuals' environment use their communication form and show that they take it seriously, they boost the individuals' status.

> At a day centre for mentally handicapped individuals a youth meeting was held once a week. One of the adolescents used manual signs, while the others were able to speak. The youth who used signs had a good understanding of speech and used 200

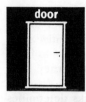

door

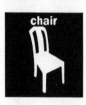

toilet

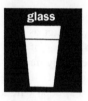

chair

glass

television

radio

bed

manual signs actively. The other youths did not use signs and had trouble understanding him at the meetings. One of the teachers therefore had to interpret for him. This led to the other youths taking what he expressed seriously, and his esteem in the group was boosted (K. Steindal, personal communication 1990).

One may use graphic signs as labels on objects in the children's environment, e.g. DOOR, TOILET, CHAIR, GLASS, TELEVISION, RADIO, BED, etc. This may make it easier for them to learn the names of things; the signs become part of the environment, and it is then easier for people to use the graphic signs when they speak to the children. One may also label cupboards and drawers containing their individual's belongings with signs that they are in the process of learning.

Teaching parents

Intervention for children has a greater and more lasting effect when the parents are included as active participants and receive proper teaching (Løvaas, 1978; Berry, 1987). This requires a cooperative effort, but in many instances either the parents are not consulted or else it is left entirely up to them to put such measures into effect. Active participation on the part of the parents does not mean that they should act as teachers for their children or assume the responsibilities of professionals. The role of parents is first and foremost to be parents, and in the case of a severely disabled child, this is a demanding enough task in itself. It may take the parents of a disabled child a considerable amount of time and energy to perform such commonplace activities with the child as dressing, washing and eating. There is often little time left for the parents and child to participate in more pleasant activities together.

The parents should be informed about what augmentative communication is, and of other peoples' experiences with using it. It is especially important to emphasise that one has not given up hope that the child will begin to speak; the aim is to enhance the possible development of speech. A natural part of the teaching is to teach the parents the communication system their child will use. This may be done either too little or too much. Parents may spend their only free evening each week in order to attend a class, struggle to find baby-sitters, etc., and find that they have learned several hundred signs at the end of one year. During the same period of time the child will have learned perhaps 10 signs. The parents may feel that this is a poor result, and they may be disappointed by the intervention of which they had great hopes and in which they had invested a lot of time.

Many of the courses that are arranged are not specifically designed for parents of autistic or mentally handicapped children, and the parents may feel that many of the signs they have learned are of little use. In such cases it may be better if the parents are taught by professionals responsible for teaching speech-impaired individuals. There are also a number of course books with sign vocabularies designed especially for children. It is unnecessary for the parents to learn a greater number of signs than the child is in the process of learning. If the child's development is rapid, this will motivate the parents to learn new signs. If the child learns to use 10 manual signs and the parents are able to use 20, then the result will be good in terms of time and energy invested.

The parents of children who learn graphic signs also need to have the system explained to them thoroughly. They need to see how the signs should be used, and preferably participate in teaching sessions at the nursery school or school. It should be emphasised that graphic signs are not merely a collection of incidental pictures but that they are the child's communication system and replace his or her lack of speech for the time being. This is especially important with simple systems such as PIC signs and PCS. Some parents begin to talk about what they see on the signs the child points to in much the same way they as though they were looking at ordinary pictures (C. Basil, personal communication 1989). This undermines the intended linguistic function of these pictures. The parents should therefore be taught how the actual communicative process takes place, and how they should use the graphic signs and ordinary pictures.

For more complex systems such as Blissymbols and Rebus signs, it appears as though many parents sabotage the use of the communication board, probably due to inadequate teaching. They feel that they do not understand their children any better than before, and choose instead to use the old form of communication where they asked the children yes—no questions. A negative attitude on the part of the parents will in many cases rub off on the children, which will generally lead to their not learning to fully utilise the linguistic tool they have at their disposal.

The parents should follow up the children's teaching. This may lead to the children being given 'homework', i.e. tasks which the parents and children are to perform at home. It is essential that the children not only learn to use new signs at nursery school or school but quickly learn to use them at home as well.

General teaching and discussion of intervention and teaching methods will not guarantee, however, that training at home is well implemented (Casey, 1978; Basil, 1986). Role-playing may be used to a certain extent, and video may also be a useful aid. The best strategy of all, however, is that of observing professionals teaching and giving practical instruction. The parents will be able to see how the children point or perform signs, which will help them to recognise their attempts to communicate in the home.

The teaching that takes place at home should not be so extensive that it encroaches upon all other activities the family enjoys. The tasks the parents are given should take into account the family's whole situation. It is easy to give the parents tasks that are too extensive, and it is not uncommon to hear criticism from professionals who do not think the parents follow up properly. It can be easy for professionals to forget that they can leave their work at the office, while the parents have the responsibility the whole time.

Teaching staff

It is essential to teach those who work with or around the individuals if the intervention is to be successful. On many occasions it is only those who show most interest, have a flair for signs, or are singled out for one reason or other, who are taught sign use. In this way it is generally only these people who are able to use signs, and know how they should react to the individuals' attempts at communication. The teaching should include everyone in contact with the individuals. Nursery school assistants may be the people who have most opportunities to communicate with the individuals, but often it is precisely this group that receives the poorest training.

The teaching of staff members should take place on a regular basis, and be aimed at all aspects of the intervention. The teaching is often inadequate, and may be limited to the learning of only a few manual signs or to a demonstration of what the graphic signs look like. It is important that the staff are taught the signs' construction and how they are formulated. Although many people feel awkward or silly pointing at graphic signs or performing manual signs, this is the easiest part of the teaching. It may be an additional advantage if the staff members do not have too much prior experience of manual signs as they will thus perform them slower and more clearly, making them easier for the individuals to perceive. In any case, it is no drawback if the manual signs are performed slowly and rather meticulously, as is often the case with novices.

In order to develop spontaneous communication, it is important that the staff members are taught to not only take the communicative initiative but also to be sensitive and respond to the individual's own attempts at communication. It is considerably more difficult to read other people's manual signs than it is to produce signs oneself. A significant part of the teaching should therefore be aimed at comprehending other people's sign use. It is particularly in everyday situations that understanding signs produced by others can be difficult. In a defined teaching situation the teacher will generally know which sign the individual is trying to perform, and will be able to respond to the sign even though it was poorly articulated.

Associations for deaf people usually have a number of videos that may be rented for teaching purposes. It is also possible to make one's own video, or perform signs that the others are supposed to guess. It is particularly useful to make a video recording of individuals performing signs, so that the members of staff can learn what the signs look like when particular individuals perform them. It can be good training to try to guess from the video which sign an individual is attempting to perform, without giving any extra clues, i.e. by turning the volume down so it is impossible to hear what the teacher is saying, by making sure that the picture is not showing the object or activity about which the individual is communicating, and taking care that the teacher does not perform the sign first.

With a number of communication aid users, it can be difficult to understand where and how they are pointing. Video recordings can be a useful means of demonstrating which method of pointing is best suited to particular individuals, and thus help to reduce the likelihood that people in the children's environment will misunderstand their pointing.

In the case of graphic signs the gloss is usually written above the sign, so it is not necessary to learn the design of each of the separate signs. All members of staff should nonetheless be given an introduction to how the system is constructed, and the reasons why specific signs are included on the individual's communication board. It is good practice for the staff members to use the signs to communicate with one another, so that they gain an insight into the system's potential and limitations. The staff should also be introduced to the more general reasons for choosing the system, and be informed about the children's expected development. This will help them to react correctly in new situations, and to take note of any significant developments.

The staff members also need to know how the individuals wish the communication to take place, e.g. whether they should guess or interpret the communication before individuals have finished saying what they want to say. The staff members must learn to become aware of their role as listeners. When using graphic signs it can be easy to lose track of what is being said, and forget to answer a question or a comment an individual has spent a long time articulating. Care should be taken to mention the difficulties that may arise from using the system, and how misunderstandings can be rectified. If the staff members know about the problems the users may encounter, it will be considerably easier to help solve them.

For users of complex systems such as Blissymbols and Rebus signs, it is essential that the staff members are familiar with single signs, the use of analogies, and basic conversational strategies. This will enable the individuals to use the system as effectively as possible, and prevent them from having to adapt their communication to a more elementary level in order to communicate with the staff members.

In addition to direct teaching and instruction, the people who are responsible for the teaching should act as models for the rest of the staff members in natural, unplanned situations. For many of the staff members, using signs will be a new experience, and a model may make it easier for them to try using what they have learned.

Individuals who use augmentative communication are often met with indifference, rejection or fear. The fact that staff members show an interest in, and an understanding of, the individual's sign system signals a positive attitude to, and respect for, the communicative form utilised by the user of augmentative language. For the expressive language group in particular, this will heighten their self-esteem. It will do no harm if a member of staff tells an individual with good language comprehension that he or she finds it difficult to master the system. An admission of this kind may make the user feel more competent, and perhaps less despairing of other people's misunderstandings and faults.

The teaching of staff members will necessarily take time and resources, but this will be money and time well spent. In special teaching programmes directed at the staff a disproportionate amount of emphasis is given to the fact that the teaching should not take too long or encroach on the time spent performing other tasks (cf. McNaughton and Light, 1989). We believe it is bad policy to save on teaching. A good educational programme will help produce competent staff who can understand and master their work. Also, this type of environment will produce the best language environment for individuals in the process of learning augmentative communication.

Overview of case studies

This chapter contains an overview of articles that deal with augmentative communication for individuals with developmental disorders. Since the aim of this chapter is to give parents and professionals access to different descriptions of augmentative communication teaching, only published articles containing studies of individuals are included. The overview contains information about the individuals' age and impairments (based on the classification made in the article), and about the communication systems that have been utilised. The full reference may be found in the list beginning on p. 234.

A considerable number of articles containing descriptions of individuals have been published, and the list given here should in no way be considered complete. However, it contains descriptions of the most common groups with developmental disorders and a need for augmentative communication, and examples of the most commonly used communication systems and teaching strategies.

Impairment groups

Autism (A)
Mental handicap (H)
Motor disability (M)
Multiple handicap (MH)
Specific language disorders (S)
Other (Oth)
Unspecified (?)

Communication systems

Blissymbols (B)
Computer-based aids (C)
Gestures (G)
Manual signs (MS)
Lexigrams (L)
Picsym (PS)
PIC signs (PIC)
Picture Communication System (PCS)
Pictures (P)
Premack's word bricks (PWB)
Rebus (R)
Script (S)
Other (Oth)
Unspecified (?)

Descriptions

Authors	Impairments	Age	System
Barrera et al., 1980	A	4	MS
Barrera and Sulzer-Azaroff, 1983	A	6, 7, 9	MS
Bedwinek, 1983	H	5	G
Bennet et al., 1986	MH	14, 14, 17	MS
Bonvillian and Nelson, 1976	A	5	MS
Bonvillian and Nelson, 1978	A	12	MS
Booth, 1978	H	15	MS
Brady and Smouse, 1978	A	6	Oth
Brookner and Murphy, 1975	H, S	13	MS, S
Bruno, 1989	M	4	P
Buzolich, 1987	M, H	7, 9, 15	MS, B, C
Carr et al., 1978	A	10–15	MS
Carr et al., 1987	A	11–16	MS
Casey, 1978	A	6, 7	MS
Clarke et al., 1986	H	6, 11, 11	MS
Clarke et al., 1988	H	5–12	MS
Coleman et al., 1980	M	44	C
Cook and Coleman, 1987	M, H	14	B, P
Culatta and Blackstone, 1980	H, MH	3, 5, 5	MS
Culp, 1989	S	8	MS
Deich and Hodges, 1977	A, H	2–20	MS, PWB
Duker and Michielsen, 1983	H	8, 12, 16	MS
Duker and Moonen, 1985	H	11, 13, 14	MS
Duker and Moonen, 1986	H	10, 12, 14	MS
Duker and Morsink, 1984	A, H	8–23	MS
Elder and Bergman, 1978	H	3–17	B
English and Prutting, 1975	Oth	1	MS
Everson and Goodwyn, 1987	M	16–19	C
Faulk, 1988	MH	9	MS, S, P, C
Fenn and Rowe, 1975	H	10–13	MS
Flensborg, 1988	M	12, 12	B, S, C
Foss, 1981	A, Oth	25, 39	MS
Foxx et al., 1988	H, MH	18, 20	MS
Fuller et al., 1983	MH	6	MS
Fulwiler and Fouts, 1976	A	5	MS
Glennen and Calculator, 1985	M, MH	5, 12	P, R, S
Goosens', 1989	M	6	PCS
Goosens' and Kraat, 1985	M, H	3, 5, 7	P, S, C
Hansen, 1986	A	6	MS
Harris, 1982	M	6, 6, 7	S, C
Hill et al., 1968	M	6	S
Hind, 1989	M	3	B, C
Hinderscheit and Reichle, 1987	MH	18	R
Hinerman et al., 1982	A	5	MS
Hobson and Duncan, 1979	H	16–57	MS
Hooper et al., 1987	MH	7	MS, B
Horner and Budd, 1985	A, H	11	MS
Hughes, 1974/75	S	7–11	PWB
Hurlbut et al., 1982	M, H	14, 16, 18	P, B
Iacono and Parsons, 1986	H	11, 13, 15	MS
Kahn, 1981	H	5–8	MS
Karlan et al., 1982	S	6–7	MS

Authors	Impairments	Age	System
Keogh et al., 1987	A, H	14, 25	MS
Kollinzas, 1983	H	20	MS
Konstantareas et al., 1977	A, H	5–9	MS
Konstantareas et al., 1979	A, H	8–10	MS
Kotkin et al., 1978	H	6, 7	MS
Kouri, 1989	H	2	MS
Lagerman and Höök, 1982	M	11	S, C
Layton and Baker, 1981	A	8	MS
Light et al., 1985	A, H	14, 14, 14	PWB
Locke and Mirenda, 1988	H	11	Oth
Luetke-Stahlman, 1985	S	5	MS
Marshall and Hegrenes, 1972	A	7	S
Maty-Laikko et al., 1989	MH	8	Oth
McDonald and Schultz, 1973	M	6	B
McEwen and Karlan, 1989	MH	3, 4	Oth
McIlvane et al., 1984	A, H	18, 27	MS
McLean and McLean, 1973	A	8, 8, 10	Oth
McNaughton and Light, 1989	M, H	27	G
Mills and Higgins,1984	M	9	R, S
Mirenda and Dattilo, 1987	H	10, 11, 12	P
Mirenda and Santogrossi, 1985	H	8	PCS
Murdock, 1978	H	15	S
Oliver and Halle, 1982	H	7	MS
Osguthorpe and Chang, 1987	M, H	11–14	R
Pecyna, 1988	H	4	R
Peters, 1973	M, MH	13	MS
Prevost, 1983	H	1	MS
Ratusnik and Ratusnik, 1974	A	10	S
Reichle and Brown, 1986	A	23	R, PIC
Reichle et al., 1984	H	15	MS
Reichle et al., 1987	A, MH	18, 18	P
Reichle and Ward, 1985	H	13	MS, S, C
Reichle and Yoder, 1985	MH	3–4	PIC
Reid and Hurlbut, 1977	M, MH	31–34	P
Remington and Clarke, 1983	A	10, 15	MS
Romski and Ruder, 1984	H	3–7	MS
Romski and Sevcik, 1989	H	18, 19	L
Romski et al., 1984	H	11–18	L
Romski et al., 1988	M, H	14–19	L
Rowe and Rapp, 1980	M, S	6, 13	MS
Salvin et al., 1977	A	5	MS
Schaeffer et al., 1977	A	4, 5, 5	MS
Schepis et al., 1982	A, H	18–21	MS
Sisson and Barrett, 1984	H	4, 7, 8	MS
Smebye, 1984	MH, H	2–7	MS, P
Smebye, 1985	MH, H	2–7	MS, P
Smebye, 1986	MH	6	MS
Smebye, 1988	MH	7	MS, C
Smeets and Striefel, 1976	H	16	MS
Smith-Lewis and Ford, 1987	S	25	MS
Sommer et al., 1988	A, MH, H	8–25	MS
Topper, 1975	H	28	MS
Trefler and Crislip, 1985	M	18	S, C
Trevinarus and Tannock, 1987	M	7, 8	B, P, S, C

Authors	Impairments	Age	System
Vanderheiden et al., 1975	M	11–16	B
Vanderheiden and Lloyd, 1986	M	7	S, C, ?
Villiers and McNaughton, 1974	A	6, 9	S
von Tetzchner, 1984a	S	3	MS
von Tetzchner, 1984b	A	5	MS
Webster et al., 1973	A, H	6	MS
Wells, 1981	H	18, 25, 26	MS
Wherry and Edwards, 1983	A	5	MS
Yorkston et al., 1989	M	36	B, PS

References

American Psychiatric Association. *Diagnostic criteria for DSM-III (Revised)*. Washington, DC: American Psychiatric Press, 1987.

Arnold, G. E. Physiology and pathology of speech and language. In R. Luchsinger and G. E. Arnold (Eds.), *Voice–Speech–Language*. Belmont, CA: Wadsworth, 1965.

Baker, B. Using images to generate speech. *Byte*, 1986, **11**, 160–168.

Baker, L. and Cantwell, D. P. Language acquisition, cognitive development, and emotional disorder in childhood. In K. E. Nelson (Ed.), *Children's language*, Volume 3. London: Erlbaum, 1982, pp. 286–321.

Balkom, L. J.M. v., Blom C. L.v. and Soede, M. *Efficient input systems for augmentative communication*. Hoensbroek: Institute for Rehabilitational Research, 1987.

Barrera, R. D., Lobato-Barrera, D. and Sulzer-Azaroff, B. A simultaneous treatment comparison of three expressive language training programs with a mute autistic child. *Journal of Autism and Developmental Disorders*, 1980, **10**, 21–37.

Barrera, R. D. and Sulzer-Azaroff, B. An alternating treatment comparison of oral and total communication training programs with echolalic autistic children. *Journal of Applied Behavior Analysis*, 1983, **16**, 379–394.

Basil, C. Social interaction and learned helplessness in nonvocal severely handicapped children. Paper presented at The Fourth Biennial Conference on Augmentative and Alternative Communication, Cardiff, 1986.

Bates, E. *The emergence of symbols*. New York: Academic Press, 1979.

Bedwinek, A. P. The use of PACE to facilitate gestural and verbal communication in a language-impaired child. *Language, Speech, and Hearing Services in Schools*, 1983, **14**, 2–6.

Bennet, D. L., Gast, D. L., Wolery, M. and Schuster, J. Time delay and system of least prompts in teaching manual sign production. *Education and Training of the Mentally Retarded*, 1986, **21**, 117–129.

Benton, A. The cognitive functioning of children with developmental dysphasia. In M. A. Wyke (Ed.), *Developmental dysphasia*. New York: Academic Press, 1977, 43–62.

Berry, J. O. Strategies for involving parents in programs for young children using augmentative and alternative communication. *Augmentative and Alternative Communication*, 1987, **3**, 90–93.

Beukelman, D. R. Evaluating the effectiveness of intervention programs. In S. W. Blackstone (Ed.), *Augmentative communication: An introduction*. Rockville, MD: American Speech and Hearing Association, 1986, pp. 423–445.

Beukelman, D. R. and Yorkston, K. M. Computer enhancement of message formulation and presentation for communication system users. *Seminars in Speech and Language*, 1984, **5**, 1–10.

Beukelman, D. R., Yorkston, K. M. and Dowden, P. A. *Augmentative communication: A casebook of clinical management*. Boston, MA: College-Hill Press, 1985.

Beukelman, D. R., Yorkston, K. M., Poblete, M. and Naranjo, C. Frequency of word occurrence in communication samples produced by adult communication aid users. *Journal of Speech and Hearing Disorders*, 1984, **49**, 360–367.

Blackstone, S. and Painter, M. Speech problems in multihandicapped children. In J. Darby (Ed.), *Speech and language evaluation in neurology: Childhood disorders*. Orlando, FL: Grune and Stratton, 1985, pp. 219–242.

Blau, A. On interaction. *Communicating Together*, 1983, **1**, 10–12.

Bliss, C. *Semantography (Blissymbolics)*. Sydney: Semantography Publications, 1965.

Bloom, L. (1973). *One word at a time*. The Hague: Mouton.

Bloomberg, K. P. and Lloyd, L. L. (1986). Graphic/aided symbols and systems: resource information. *Communication Outlook*, 1986, **7**, 24–30.

Bo-enheden M-huset. *Hva sker der i M-Huset???* Copenhagen: Københavns Amtskommune, 1986.

Bondurant, J. L., Romeo, D. J. and Kretschmer, R. Language behaviors of mothers of children with normal and delayed language. *Language, Speech, and Hearing Services in Schools*, 1983, **14**, 233–242.

Bonvillian, J. D. and Nelson, K. E. Sign language acquisition in a mute autistic boy. *Journal of Speech and Hearing Disorders*, 1976, **41**, 339–347.

Bonvillian, J. D. and Nelson, K. E. Development of sign language in language-handicapped individuals. In P. Siple (Ed.), *Understanding language through sign language research*. New York: Academic Press, 1978, 187–212.

Bonvillian, J. D., Orlansky, M. D. and Novack, L. L. Early sign language acquisition and its relation to cognitive and motor development. Paper presented at the Second International Symposium on Sign Language Research, Bristol, July 1981.

Booth, T. Early receptive language training for the severely and profoundly retarded. *Language, Speech, and Hearing Services in Schools*, 1978, **9**, 142–150.

Bottorf, L. and DePape, D. Initiating communication systems for severely speech-impaired persons. *Topics in Language Disorders*, 1982, **2**, 55–71.

Brady, D. O. and Smouse, A. D. A simultaneous comparison of three methods for language training with an autistic child. *Journal of Autism and Childhood Schizophrenia*, 1978, **8**, 271–279.

Braine, M. D.S. The ontogeny of English phrase structure: The first phase. *Language*, 1963, **39**, 1–14.

Broch, I. and Jahr, E. H. *Russenorsk – et pidginspråk i Norge*. Oslo: Novus, 1981.

Brookner, S. P. and Murphy, N. O. The use of a total communication approach with a nondeaf child: A case study. *Language, Speech, and Hearing Services in Schools*, 1975, 6, 313–139.

Brown, R. Why are signed languages easier to learn than spoken languages? Paper presented at the National Symposium on Sign Language Research and Teaching, Chicago, 1977.

Bruno, J. Customizing a Minspeak system for a preliterate child: A case example. *Augmentative and Alternative Communication*, 1989, 5, 89–100.

Bruno, J. and Bryen, D. N. The impact of modelling on physically disabled nonspeaking children's communication. Paper presented at the Fourth Biennial Conference on Augmentative and Alternative Communication, Cardiff, 1986.

Bryen, D. N. and Joyce, D. G. Language intervention with the severely handicapped: A decade of research. *Journal of Special Education*, 1985, 19, 7–39.

Burkhart, L. J. *Using computers and speech synthesis to facilitate communicative interaction with young and/or severely handicapped children.* College Park, MD: Burkhart, 1987.

Buzolich, M. J. Children in transition: Implementing augmentative communication systems with severely speech-handicapped children. *Seminars in Speech and Language*, 1987, 8, 199–213.

Byler, J. K. The Makaton vocabulary: An analysis based on recent research. *British Journal of Special Education*, 1985, 12, 113–129.

Calculator, S. N. and Delaney, D. Comparison of nonspeaking and speaking mentally retarded adults' clarification strategies. *Journal of Speech and Hearing Disorders*, 1986, 51, 252–259.

Calculator, S. and Dollaghan, C. The use of communication boards in a residential setting: An evaluation. *Journal of Speech and Hearing Disorders*, 1982, 47, 281–287.

Calculator, S. and Luchko, C. D'A. Evaluating the effectiveness of a communication board training program. *Journal of Speech and Hearing Disorders*, 1983, 48, 185–191.

Caparulo, B. K. and Cohen, D. J. Cognitive structures, language, and emerging social competence in autistic and aphasic children. *Journal of the American Academy of Child Psychiatry*, 1977, 16, 620–645.

Carlson, F. A format for selecting vocabulary for the nonspeaking child. *Language, Speech, and Hearing Services in Schools*, 1981, 12, 240–145.

Carr, E. G. Language acquisition in developmentally disabled children. *Annals of Child Development*, 1985, 2, 49–76.

Carr, E. G. Tegnspråk. In O. I. Løvaas, *Opplæring av utviklingshemmede barn.* Oslo: Gyldendal, 1988, pp. 177–186.

Carr, E. G., Binkoff, J. A., Kologinsky, E. and Eddy, M. Acquisition of sign language by autistic children. I: Expressive labelling. *Journal of Applied Behavior Analysis*, 1978, 11, 489–501.

Carr, E. G., Kologinsky, E. and Leff-Simon, S. Acquisition of sign language by autistic children. III: Generalized descriptive phrases. *Journal of Autism and Developmental Disorders*, 1987, 17, 217–229.

Carrier, J. K. Nonspeech noun usage training with severely and profoundly retarded children. *Journal of Speech and Hearing Research*, 1974, 17, 510–517.

Carrier, J. K. and Peak, T. *NONSLIP (non-speech language initiation program)*. Kansas City, MO: H. and H. Enterprise, 1975.

Casey, L. O. Development of communicative behavior in autistic children: A parent program using manual signs. *Journal of Autism and Childhood Schizophrenia*, 1978, **8**, 45–59.

Chapman, R. S. and Miller, J. F. Analyzing language and communication in the child. In R. L. Schiefelbusch (Ed.), *Nonspeech language and communication*. Baltimore, MD: University Park Press, 1980, pp. 159–196.

Clark, C. R. Learning words using traditional orthography and the symbols of Rebus, Bliss and Carrier. *Journal of Speech and Hearing Disorders*, 1981, **46**, 191–196.

Clark, C. R. A close look at the standard Rebus system and Blissymbolics. *Journal of the Association for Persons with Severe Handicaps*, 1984, **9**, 37–48.

Clark, E. V. Convention and contrast in acquiring the lexicon. In T. B. Seiler and W. Wannenmacher (Eds.), *Concept development and the development of word meaning*. New York: Springer-Verlag, 1983.

Clark, R. Theory and method in child-language research: Are we assuming too much? In S. Kuczaj, II (Ed.), *Language development, Volume 1: Syntax and semantics*. Hillsdale, NJ: Erlbaum, 1982, pp. 1–36.

Clarke, S., Remington, B. and Light, P. An evaluation of the relationship between receptive speech skills and expressive signing. *Journal of Applied Behavior Analysis*, 1986, **19**, 231–239.

Clarke, S., Remington, B. and Light, P. The role of referential speech in sign learning by mentally retarded children: A comparison of total communication and sign-alone training. *Journal of Applied Behavior Analysis*, 1988, **21**, 419–426.

Coleman, C. L., Cook, A. M. and Meyers, L. S. Assessing non-oral clients for assistive communication devices. *Journal of Speech and Hearing Research*, 1980, **45**, 515–526.

Conway, N. My perceptions of communication aids. Paper presented at the Fourth Biennial Conference on Augmentative and Alternative Communication, Cardiff, 1986.

Cook, A. M. and Coleman, C. L. Selecting augmentative communication systems by matching client skills and needs to system characteristics. *Seminars in Speech and Language*, 1987, **8**, 153–167.

Cooper, J. M. and Griffiths, P. Treatment and prognosis. In M. A. Wyke (Ed.), *Developmental dysphasia*. New York: Academic Press, 1977, pp. 159–176.

Cregan, A. *Sigsymbol dictionary*. Cambridge: LDA, 1982.

Cregan, A. and LLoyd, L. L. *Sigsymbol dictionary: American edition*. West Lafayette, IN: Purdue University Press, 1984.

Culatta, B. and Blackstone, S. A program to teach non-oral communication symbols to multiply handicapped children. *Journal of Childhood Communication Disorders*, 1980, **1**, 29–55.

Culp, D. M. Communication interactions – nonspeaking children using augmentative systems and their mothers. Unpublished manuscript, 1982.

Culp, D. M. Developmental apraxia and augmentative or alternative communication – a case example. *Augmentative and Alternative Communication*, 1989, **5**, 27–34.

Dalhof, F. *Forstår han hvad man sier?* Fredrikshavn: Dafolo Forlag, 1986.

Deacon, J. *Tongue tied.* London: Spastics Society, 1974.

Deich, R. F. and Hodges, P. M. *Language without speech.* London: Souvenir Press, 1977.

Deich, R. F. and Hodges, P. M. Teaching nonvocal communications to nonverbal retarded children. *Behavior Modification*, 1982, 6, 200–228.

Dennis, R., Reichle, J., Williams, W. and Vogelsberg, R. T. Motoric factors influencing the selection of vocabulary for sign production programs. *Journal of the Association for Persons with Severe Handicaps*, 1982, 7, 20–32.

Dixon, L. S. A functional analysis of photo-object matching skills of severely retarded adolescents. *Journal of Applied Behavior Analysis*, 1981, 14, 465–478.

Doherty, J. E. The effect of sign characteristics on sign acquisition and retention: An integrative review of the literature. *Augmentative and Alternative Communication*, 1985, 1, 108–121.

Downing, J. (Ed.), *Comparative reading.* New York: MacMillan, 1973.

Duker, P. C. and Michielsen, H. M. Cross-setting generalization of manual signs to verbal instructions with severely retarded children. *Applied Research in Mental Retardation*, 1983, 4, 29–40.

Duker, P. C. and Moonen, X. M. A program to increase manual signs with severely/profoundly mentally retarded students in natural environments. *Applied Research in Mental Retardation*, 1985, 6, 147–158.

Duker, P. C. and Moonen, X. M. The effect of two procedures on spontaneous signing with Down's syndrome children. *Journal of Mental Deficiency Research*, 1986, 30, 335–364.

Duker, P. C. and Morsink, H. Acquisition and cross-setting generalization of manual signs with severely retarded individuals. *Journal of Applied Behavior Analysis*, 1984, 17, 93–103.

Elder, P. S. and Bergman, J. S. Visual symbol communication instruction with nonverbal, multiply-handicapped individuals. *Mental Retardation*, 1978, 16, 107–112.

English, S. T. and Prutting, C. A. Teaching American sign language to a normally hearing infant with tracheostenosis. *Clinical Pediatrics*, 1975, 14, 1141–1145.

Everson, J. M. and Goodwyn, R. A comparison of the use of adaptive microswitches by students with cerebral palsy. *American Journal of Occupational Therapy*, 1987, 41, 739–744.

Faulk, J. P. Touch Talker: A case study. *Communication Outlook*, 1988, 10, 8–11.

Fenn, G. and Rowe, J. A. An experiment in manual communication. *British Journal of Disorders of Communication*, 1975, 10, 3–16.

Ferguson, C. A. Learning to pronounce: The earliest stages of phonological development in the child. In F. D. Minifie and L. L. Lloyd (Eds.), *Communicative and cognitive abilities – Early behavioral assessment.* Baltimore, MD: University Park Press, 1978, pp. 273–297.

Ferguson, C. A. and Debose, C. E. Simplified registers, broken language, and pidginization. In A. Valman (Ed.), *Pidgin and Creole linguistics.* Bloomington, IN: Indiana University Press, 1977, pp. 99–125.

Fishman, I. R. *Electronic communication aids and techniques: Selection and use.* San Diego, CA: College Hill, 1987.

Flensborg, C. *Snak med mig.* København: Socialstyrelsen, 1988.

Foss, N. E. Tegnspråkopplæring av autister og psykisk utviklings-hemmede. Dissertation, Universitetet i Oslo, 1981.

Foxx, R. M., Kyle, M. S., Faw, G. D. and Bittle, R. G. Cues–pause-point training and simultaneous communication to teach the use of signed labeling repertoires. *American Journal of Mental Retardation*, 1988, 93, 305–311.

Fristoe, M. and Lloyd, L. L. Planning an initial expressive sign lexicon for persons with severe communication impairment. *Journal of Speech and Hearing Disorders*, 1980, 45, 170–180.

Frith, U. *Autism. Explaining the enigma.* Oxford: Blackwell, 1989.

Fry, D. B. The development of the phonological system in the normal and the deaf child. In F. Smith and G. A. Miller (Eds.), *The genesis of language.* London: MIT Press, 1966, pp. 187–206.

Fuller, P., Newcombe, F. and Ounsted, C. Late language development in a child unable to recognize or produce speech sounds. *Archives of Neurology*, 1983, 40, 165–169.

Fuller, D. R. and Lloyd, L. L. A study of physical and semantic characteristics of a graphic symbol system as predictors of perceived complexity. *Augmentative and Alternative Communication*, 1987, 3, 26–35.

Fulwiler, R. L. and Fouts, R. S. Acquisition of American sign language by a noncommunicating autistic child. *Journal of Autism and Childhood Schizophrenia*, 1976, 6, 43–51.

Fundudis, T., Kolvin, I. and Garside, R. (Eds.), *Speech retarded and deaf children: Their psychological development.* London: Academic Press, 1979.

Gibson, D. *Down's syndrome: The psychology of mongolism.* Cambridge: Cambridge University Press, 1978.

Glennen, S. L. and Calculator, S. N. Training functional communication board use: a pragmatic approach. *Augmentative and Alternative Communication*, 1985, 1, 134–142.

Goosens', C. A. The relative iconicity and learnability of verb referents represented in Blissymbolics, Rebus symbols, and manual signs: An investigation with moderately retarded individuals. Doctoral dissertation, Purdue University, IN, 1983.

Goosens', C. A. Aided communication intervention before assessment: A case study of a child with cerebral palsy. *Augmentative and Alternative Communication*, 1989, 3, 14–26.

Goosens', C. A. and Crain, S. S. Overview of nonelectronic eye-gaze communication techniques. *Augmentative and Alternative Communication*, 1987, 3, 77–89.

Goosens', C. A. and Kraat, A. Technology as a tool for conversation and language learning for the physically disabled. *Topics in Language Disorders*, 1985, 6, 56–70.

Grandin, T. An autistic person's view of holding therapy. *Communication*, 1989, 23, 75–78.

Griffith, P. L. and Robinson, J. H. A comparative and normative study of the iconicity of signs rated by three groups. *American Annals of the Deaf*, 1981, 126, 440–449.

Guillaume, P. *Imitation in children.* Chicago: Chicago University Press, 1971.

Hagberg, B. Rett syndrome: Swedish approach to analysis of prevalence and cause. *Brain and Development*, 1985, 7, 277–280.

Hagberg, B. and Witt-Engström, I. Rett syndrome: A suggested staging system for describing impairment profile with increasing age toward adolescence. *American Journal of Medical Genetics*, 1986, **24**, 47–59.

Hagen, C., Porter, W. and Brink. J. Nonverbal communication: An alternate mode of communication for the child with severe cerebral palsy. *Journal of Speech and Hearing Disorders*, 1973, **38**, 448–455.

Hagtvet, B. and Lillestøln, R. *Reynells språktest*. Oslo: Universitetsforlaget, 1985.

Halle, J. W., Alpert, C. L. and Anderson, S. R. Natural environment language assessment and intervention with severely impaired preschoolers. *Topics in Early Childhood Special Education*, 1984, **4**, 36–56.

Hansen, E. M. Jon lærer tegn. Dissertation, Statens Spesiallærerhøgkole, 1986.

Hardy, J. C. *Cerebral palsy*. Englewood Cliffs, NJ: Prentice-Hall, 1983.

Harris, D. Communicative interaction processes involving nonvocal physically handicapped children. *Topics in Language Disorders*, 1982, **2**, 21–37.

Helgevold, K. A. Situasjonsvariasjon ved elektiv mutisme. Dissertation, Universitetet i Oslo, 1989.

Hermelin, B. A. and O'Connor, N. *Psychological experiments with autistic children*. Oxford: Pergamon Press, 1970.

Higgins, J. and Mills, J. Communication training in real environments. In S. W. Blackstone (Ed.), *Augmentative communication: An introduction*. Rockville, MD: American Speech and Hearing Association, 1986, pp. 345–352.

Hill, S. D., Campagna, J., Long, D., Munch, J. and Naecker, S. An explorative study of the use of two response keyboards as a means of communication for the severely handicapped child. *Perceptual and Motor Skills*, 1968, **26**, 699–704.

Hind, M. Synrel: Programs to teach sequencing of Blissymbols. *Communication Outlook*, 1989, **10**, 6–9.

Hinderscheit, L. R. and Reichle, J. Teaching direct select color encoding to an adolescent with multiple handicaps. *Augmentative and Alternative Communication*, 1987, **3**, 137–142.

Hinerman, P. S., Jenson, W. R., Walker, G. R. and Petersen, P. B. Positive practice overcorrection combined with additional procedures to teach signed words to an autistic child. *Journal of Autism and Developmental Disorders*, 1982, **12**, 253–263.

Hobson, P. A. and Duncan, P. Sign learning and profoundly retarded people. *Mental Retardation*, 1979, **17**, 33–37.

Hodges, P. M. and Deich, R. F. Teaching an artificial language system to nonverbal retardates. *Behavior Modification*, 1978, **2**, 489–509.

Hodges, P. M. and Schwethelm, B. A comparison of the effectiveness of graphic symbol and manual sign training with profoundly retarded children. *Applied Psycholinguistics*, 1984, **5**, 223–253.

Hooper, J., Connell, T. M. and Flett, P. J. Blissymbols and manual signs: A multimodal approach to intervention in a case of multiple disability. *Augmentative and Alternative Communication*, 1987, **3**, 68–76.

Horner, R. H. and Budd, C. M. Acquisition of manual sign use: Collateral reduction of maladaptive behavior, and factors limiting generalization. *Education and Training of the Mentally Retarded*, 1985, **20**, 39–47.

Hughes, J. Acquisition of a non-vocal `language' by aphasic children. *Cognition*, 1974/75, **3**, 41–55.

Hurlbut, B. I., Iwata, B. A. and Green, J. D. Nonvocal language acquisition in adolescents with severe physical disabilities: Blissymbol vs. iconic stimulus formats. *Journal of Applied Behavior Analysis*, 1982, **15**, 241–258.

Hupp, S. C. Use of multiple exemplars in object concept training: How many are sufficient? *Analysis and Intervention in Developmental Disabilities*, 1986, **6**, 305–317.

Iacono, T. A. and Parsons, C. L. A comparison of techniques for teaching signs to intellectually disabled individuals using an alternating treatment design. *Australian Journal of Human Communication Disorders*, 1986, **14**, 23–34.

Ingram, T. T.S. Specific disorders of speech in childhood. *Brain*, 1959, **82**, 450–467.

Ingram, T. T.S. Speech disorders in childhood. In E. H. Lenneberg and E. Lenneberg (Eds.), *Foundations of Language Development*. New York: Academic Press, 1975, pp. 195–261.

Johannessen, A.-M. and Preus, R. F. Brytere for funksjonshemmede, del 1. *CP-Bladet*, 1989a, **35**, 16–18.

Johannessen, A.-M. and Preus, R. F. Brytere for funksjonshemmede, del 2. *CP-Bladet*, 1989b, **35**, 18–23.

Johansson, I. Tecken – en genväg till tal. *Down Syndrom: Språk ock tal*, 1987, publikation nr. 28.

Johnson, R. *The picture communication symbols*. Solana Beach, CA: Mayer-Johnson, 1981.

Johnson, R. *The picture communication symbols – Book II*. Solana Beach, CA: Mayer-Johnson, 1985.

Jones, K. A Rebus system of non-fade visual language. *Child: Care, Health and Development*, 1979, **5**, 1–7.

Kahn, J. V. A comparison of sign and verbal language training with nonverbal retarded children. *Journal of Speech and Hearing Research*, 1981, **24**, 113–119.

Karlan, G. R., Brenn-White, B., Lentz, A., Hodur, P., Egger, D. and Frankoff, D. Establishing generalized, productive verb–noun phrase usage in a manual language system with moderately handicapped children. *Journal of Speech and Hearing Disorders*, 1982, **47**, 31–42.

Keogh, D., Whitman, T., Beeman, D., Halligan, K. and Starzynski, T. Teaching interactive signing in a dialogue situation to mentally retarded individuals. *Research in Developmental Disabilities*, 1987, **8**, 39–53.

Kiernan, C. and Reid, B. *Pre-verbal communication schedule*. Windsor: NFER-Nelson, 1987.

Kiernan, C., Reid, B. and Jones, L. *Signs and symbols*. London: Heinemann, 1982.

Kirk, S.A., McCarthy, J.J. and Kirk, W.D. *Illinois Test of Psycholinguistic Ability*. Urbana, IL: University of Illinois Press, 1968.

Kirman, B. H. Mental Retardation: Medical aspects. In M. Rutter and L. Hersov (Eds.), *Child and adolescent psychiatry*. Oxford: Blackwell, 1985, pp. 650–660.

Klima, E. and Bellugi, U. *The signs of language*. London: Harvard University Press, 1979.

Kohl, F. L. Effects of motoric requirements on the acquisition of manual sign responses by severely handicapped students. *American Journal of Mental Deficiency*, 1981, **85**, 396–403.

Koke, S. and Neilson, J. The effect of auditory feedback on the spelling of nonspeaking physically disabled individuals who use microcomputers. Unpublished manuscript, University of Toronto, 1987.

Kollinzas, G. The communication record: Sharing information to promote sign language generalization. *Journal of the Association for Persons with Severe Handicaps*, 1983, **8**, 49–55.

Konstantareas, M. M., Oxman, J. and Webster, C. D. Simultaneous communication with autistic and other severely dysfunctional nonverbal children. *Journal of Communication Disorders*, 1977, **10**, 267–282.

Konstantareas, M. M., Webster, C. D. and Oxman, J. Manual language acquisition and its influence on other areas of functioning in four autistic and autistic-like children. *Journal of Child Psychology and Psychiatry*, 1979, **20**, 337–350.

Kose, G., Beilin, H. and O'Connor, J. M. Children's comprehension of actions depicted in photographs. Developmental Psychology, 1983, **19**, 636–643.

Kotkin, R. A., Simpson, S. B. and Desanto, D. The effect of sign language on the picture naming in two retarded girls possessing normal hearing. *Journal of Mental Deficiency Research*, 1978, **22**, 19–25.

Kouri, T. How manual sign acquisition relates to the development of spoken language: A case study. *Language, Speech, and Hearing Services in Schools*, 1989, **20**, 50–62.

Kraat, A. *Communication interaction between aided and natural speakers*. Toronto: Canadian Rehabilitation Council for the Disabled, 1985.

Lagergren, J. Children with motor handicaps. *Acta Paediatrica Scandinavia*, 1981, supplement 289.

Lagerman, U. and Höök, O. Communication aids for patients with dys/anathria. *Scandinavian Journal of Rehabilitational Medicine*, 1982, **14**, 155–158.

Lane, H. *When the mind hears*. London: Penguin, 1984.

Lahey, M. and Bloom, L. Planning a lexicon: Which words to teach first. *Journal of Speech and Hearing Disorders*, 1977, **42**, 340–350.

Layton, T. L. and Baker, P. S. Description of semantic–syntactic relations in an autistic child. *Journal of Autism and Developmental Disorders*, 1981, **11**, 385–399.

Lenneberg, E. H. *Biological foundations of language*. New York: Wiley, 1967.

Leonard, L. B. Facilitating linguistic skills in children with specific language impairment. *Applied Psycholinguistics*, 1981, **2**, 89–118.

Light, J. *The communicative interaction patterns of young nonspeaking physically disabled children and their primary caregivers*. Toronto: Blissymbolics Communication Institute, 1985.

Light, J., Collier, B. and Parnes, P. Communicative interaction between young nonspeaking physically disabled children and their primary caregivers: Part 1 – Discourse patterns. *Augmentative and Alternative Communication*, 1985, **1**, 74–83.

Lindberg, B. *Retts syndrom – en kartlegging av psykologiske och pedagogiska erfarenheter i Sverige.* Stockholm: Högskolan för lärarutbildning i Stockholm, 1987.

Lock, A. *The guided reinvention of language.* London: Academic Press, 1980.

Locke, P. A. and Mirenda, P. A computer-supported approach for a child with severe communication, visual, and cognitive impairments: A case study. *Augmentative and Alternative Communication,* 1988, 4, 15–22.

Lossiusutvalget. Levekår for psykisk utviklingshemmede. *NOU,* 1985, Nr. 34.

Løvaas, O. I. Parents as therapists. In M. Rutter and E. Schopler (Eds.), *Autism: A reappraisal of concepts and treatment.* London: Plenum Press, 1978, pp. 369–378.

Løvaas, O. I., Koegel, R. L. and Schreibman, L. Stimulus overselectivity in autism: A review of research. *Psychological Bulletin,* 1979, 86, 1236–1254.

Lucariello, J. Concept formation and its relation to word learning and use in the second year of life. *Journal of Child Language,* 1987, 14, 309–332.

Luetke-Stahlman, B. Using single design to verify language learning in a hearing, aphasic boy. *Sign Language Studies,* 1985, 46, 73–86.

Luftig, R. L. An analysis of initial sign lexicons as a function of eight learnability variables. *Journal of the Association for Persons with Severe Handicaps,* 1984, 9, 193–200.

Luria, A. R. *The mind of a mnemonist.* London: Jonathan Cape, 1969.

Lyon, S. R. and Ross, L. E. Comparison scan training and the matching and scanning performance of severely and profoundly mentally retarded students. *Applied Research in Mental Retardation,* 1984, 5, 439–449.

Madge, N. and Fassam, M. *Ask the children.* London: Batsford, 1982.

Magnusson, M. and Lundman, M. Datorkonferenser för talhandikappade. Paper presented at the Forskningskonferansen ´Människa–Miljö–Handikapp', Örebro, 1987.

Maharaj, S. C. *Pictogram ideogram communication.* Regina, Canada: The George Reed Foundation for the Handicapped, 1980.

Marshall, N. R. and Hegrenes, J. The use of written language as a communication system for an autistic child. *Journal of Speech and Hearing Disorders,* 1972, 37, 258–261.

Martinsen, H. Biologiske forutsetninger for kulturalisering. *Tidsskrift for Norsk Psykologforening, Monografiserien,* 1980, 6, 122–129.

Martinsen, H., Nordeng, H. and von Tetzchner, S. *Tegnspråk.* Oslo: Universitetsforlaget, 1985.

Matas, J. A., Mathy-Laikko, P., Beukelman, D. R and Legresley, K. Identifying the nonspeaking population. *Augmentative and Alternative Communication,* 1985, 1, 17–31.

Mathy-Laikko, P., Iacono, T., Ratcliff, A., Villarruel, F., Yoder, D. and Vanderheiden, G. Teaching a child with multiple disabilities to use a tactile augmentative communication device. *Augmentative and Alternative Communication,* 1989, 5, 249–256.

McDonald, E. T. and Schultz, A. R. Communication boards for cerebral-palsied children. *Journal of Speech and Hearing Disorders,* 1973, 38, 73–88.

McEwen, I. R. and Karlan, G. R. Assessment of effects of position on communication board access by individuals with cerebral palsy. *Augmentative and Alternative Communication,* 1989, 5, 235–242.

McIlvane, W. J., Bass, R. W., O'Brien, J. M., Gerovac B. J. and Stoddard, L. T. Spoken and signed naming of foods after receptive exclusion training in severe retardation. *Applied Research in Mental Retardation*, 1984, 5, 1–27.

McLean, L. P. and McLean, J. E. A language training program for nonverbal autistic children. *Journal of Speech and Hearing Disorders*, 1973, 39, 186–193.

McNaughton, D. and Light, J. Teaching facilitators to support the communication skills of an adult with severe cognitive disabilities: A case study. *Augmentative and Alternative Communication*, 1989, 5, 35–41.

McNaughton, S. and Kates, B. Visual symbols: Communication system for the pre-reading physically handicapped child. Paper presented at the American Association on Mental Deficiency Annual Meeting, Toronto, 1974.

McNaughton, S. and Kates, B. The application of Blissymbolics. In R. L. Schiefelbusch (Ed.), *Nonspeech language and communication: Analysis and interventions.* Baltimore, MD: University Park Press, 1980, pp. 303–321.

Miller, M. S. Sign iconicity: single-sign receptive vocabulary skills of nonsigning hearing preschoolers. *Journal of Communication Disorders*, 1987, 20, 359–365.

Mills, J. and Higgins, J. An environmental approach to delivery of microcomputer-based and other communication systems. *Seminars in Speech and Language*, 1984, 5, 35–45.

Mirenda, P. and Dattilo, J. Instructional techniques in alternative communication for students with severe intellectual handicap. *Augmentative and Alternative Communication*, 1987, 3, 143–152.

Mirenda, P. and Santogrossi, J. A prompt-free strategy to teach pictoral communication system use. *Augmentative and Alternative Communication*, 1985, 1, 143–150.

Morley, M. E. *The development and disorders of speech in childhood.* Edinburgh: Churchill Livingstone, 1972.

Morningstar, D. Blissymbol communication: Comparison of interaction with naive vs. experienced listeners. Unpublished manuscript, University of Toronto, 1981.

Morris, S. E. Communication/interaction development at mealtimes for the multiple handicapped child: Implications for the use of augmentative communication systems. *Language, Speech, and Hearing Services in Schools*, 1981, 12, 216–232.

Murdock, J. Y. A non-oral expressive communication program for a nonverbal retardate. *Journal of Childhood Communication Disorders*, 1978, 2, 18–25.

Nadel, L. (Ed.) *The psychobiology of Down Syndrome.* London: MIT Press, 1988.

Oliver, C. B. and Halle, J. W. Language training in the everyday environment. *Journal of the Association for Persons with Severe Handicaps*, 1982, 8, 50–62.

Osguthorpe, R. T. and Chang, L. L. Computerized symbol processors for individuals with severe communication disabilities. *Journal of Special Education Technology*, 1987, 8, 43–54.

Pecyna, P. M. Rebus symbol communication training with a severely handicapped preschool child: A case study. *Language, Speech, and Hearing Services in Schools*, 1988, 19, 128–143.

Peters, L. J. Sign language stimulus vocabulary learning of a brain-injured child. *Sign Language Research*, 1973, **3**, 116–118.

Petretic, P. A. and Tweeneny, R. D. Does comprehension precede the production? The development of children's responses to telegraphic sentences of varying grammatical adequacy. *Journal of Child Language*, 1977, **4**, 201–209.

Piaget, J. and Inhelder, B. *The psychology of the child*. London: Routledge and Kegan Paul, 1969.

Pictogrammer. Oslo: Aventura forlag, 1989.

Pierce, C. S. *Collected papers*. Cambridge: Harvard University Press, 1931.

Premack, D. Language in a chimpanzee? *Science*, 1971, **172**, 808–822.

Prevost, P. I. Using the Makaton vocabulary in early language learning with a Down's baby. *Mental Handicap*, 1983, **11**, 28–29.

Prinz, P.M. and Prinz, E.A. Acquisition of ASL and spoken English by a hearing child of a deaf mother and a hearing father: phase I – Early lexical development. *Papers and Reports on Child Language Development*, 1979, **17**, 136–146

Prinz, P.M. and Prinz, E.A. Acquisition of ASL and spoken English by a hearing child of a deaf mother and a hearing father: phase II – Early combinatorial patterns. *Sign Language Studies*, 1981, **30**, 78–88

Ratusnik, C. M. and Ratusnik, D. L. A comprehensive communication approach for a ten-year-old nonverbal autistic child. *American Journal of Orthopsychiatry*, 1974, **44**, 396–403.

Reichle, J., Barrett, C., Tetlie, R. R. and McQuarter, R. J. The effect of prior intervention to establish generalized requesting on the acquisition of object labels. *Augmentative and Alternative Communication*, 1987, **3**, 3–11.

Reichle, J. and Brown, L. Teaching the use of a multipage direct selection communication board to an adult with autism. *Journal of the Association for Persons with Severe Handicaps*, 1986, **11**, 68–73.

Reichle, J. and Karlan, G. The selection of an augmentative communication system in communication intervention: A critique of decision rules. *Journal of the Association for Persons with Severe Handicaps*, 1985, **10**, 146–156.

Reichle, J., Rogers, N. and Barrett, C. Establishing pragmatic discriminations among the communicative functions of requesting, rejecting, and commenting in an adolescent. *Journal of the Association for Persons with Severe Handicaps*, 1984, **9**, 31–36.

Reichle, J. and Ward, M. Teaching discriminative use of an encoding electronic communication device and Signing Exact English to a moderately handicapped child. *Language, Speech, and Hearing Services in Schools*, 1985, **16**, 58–63.

Reichle, L. and Yoder, D. E. Communication use in severely handicapped learners. *Language, Speech, and Hearing Services in Schools*, 1985, **16**, 146–157.

Reid, D. H. and Hurlbut, R. Teaching nonvocal communication skills to multihandicapped retarded adults. *Journal of Applied Behavior Analysis*, 1977, **10**, 591–603.

Remington, B. and Clarke, S. Acquisition of expressive signing by autistic children: An evaluation of the relative effects of simultaneous communication and sign-alone training. *Journal of Applied Behavior Analysis*, 1983, **16**, 3154–3328.

Remington, B. and Light, P. Some problems in the evaluation of research on non-oral communication systems. *Advances in Mental Handicaps*, 1983, **2**, 69–94.

Reynell, J. *Renell developmental language scales*. London: National Foundation for Educational Research, 1969.

Rimland, B. The differentiation of childhood psychosis: an analysis of checklists for 2,218 psychotic children. *Journal of Autism and Childhood Schizophrenia*, 1971, **1**, 161–174.

Romski, M. A. and Ruder, K. F. Effect of speech and speech and sign instruction on oral language learning and generalization of action+object combinations by Down's syndrome children. *Journal of Speech and Hearing Research*, 1984, **49**, 293–302.

Romski, M. A. and Sevcik, R. A. An analysis of visual-graphic symbol meanings for two nonspeaking adults with severe mental retardation. *Augmentative and Alternative Communication*, 1989, **5**, 109–114.

Romski, M. A., Sevcik, R. A. and Pate, J. L. Establishment of symbolic communication in persons with severe retardation. *Journal of Speech and Hearing Disorders*, 1988, **53**, 94–107.

Romski, M. A., Sevcik, R. A., Pate J. L. and Rumbaugh, D. M. Discrimination of Lexigrams and traditional orthography by nonspeaking severely mentally retarded children. *American Journal of Mental Deficiency*, 1985, **90**, 185–189.

Romski, M. A., White, R. A., Millen, C. E. and Rumbaugh, D. M. Effects of computer-keyboard teaching on the symbolic communication of severely retarded persons: Five case studies. *Psychological Record*, 1984, **34**, 39–54.

Rosenblum, S. M., Arick, J. R., Krug, D. A. Stubbs, E. G., Young, N. B. and Pelson, R. O. Auditory brainstem evoked responses in autistic children. *Journal of Autism and Childhood Disorders*, 1980, **10**, 215–225.

Rostad, A. M. Erfaringer med tegnopplæring av psykisk utviklingshemmede småbarn. Unpublished manuscript, 1989.

Rowe, J. A. and Rapp, D. L. Tantrums: Remediation through communication. *Child: Care, Health, and Development*, 1980, **6**, 197–208.

Rutter, M. Infantile autism and other pervasive developmental disorders. In M. Rutter and L. Hersov (Eds.), *Child and adolescent psychiatry*. Oxford: Blackwell, 1985, pp. 545–566.

Ryan, J. Early language development: Towards a communication analysis. In M. P. M. Richards (Ed.), *The integration of a child into a social world*. London: Cambridge University Press, 1974, 185–213.

Ryan, J. The silence of stupidity. In J. Morton and J. C. Marshall (Eds.), *Psycholinguistic series, Vol 1. Developmental and pathological*. London: Elek Science, 1977, pp. 99–124.

Salvin, A., Routh, D. K., Foster, R. E. Jr. and Lovejoy, K. M. Acquisition of modified American Sign Language by a mute autistic child. *Journal of Autism and Childhood Schizophrenia*, 1977, **7**, 359–371.

Schaeffer, B., Kollinzas, G., Musil, A. and McDowell, P. Spontaneous verbal language for autistic children through signed speech. *Sign Language Studies*, 1977, **17**, 387–328.

Schaeffer, B., Musil, A. and Kollinzas, G. *Total communication*. Champaign, IL: Research Press, 1980.

Schank, R. C. and Abelson, R. P. *Scripts, plans, goals, and understanding*. Hillsdale, NJ: Erlbaum, 1977.

Schepis, M. M., Reid, D. H., Fitzgerald, J. R., Faw, G. D., Pol, A. v.d. and Welty, P. A. A program for increasing manual signing by autistic and profoundly retarded youth within the daily environment. *Journal of Behavior Analysis*, 1982, **15**, 363–379.

Schopler, E., Reichler, R. J., DeVellis, R. F. and Daly, K. Toward objective classification of childhood autism: Childhood Autism Rating Scale (CARS). *Journal of Autism and Developmental Disorders*, 1980, **10**, 91–103.

Schjølberg, S. Forståelighet av talen til barn med språkvansker. Dissertation, Universitetet i Oslo, 1984.

Shane, H. C. and Bashir, A. S. Election criteria for the adoption of an augmentative communication system: Preliminary considerations. *Journal of Speech and Hearing Disorders*, 1981, **45**, 408–414.

Shane, H. C. and Cohen, C. G. A discussion of communicative strategies and patterns by nonspeaking persons. *Language, Speech, and Hearing Services in Schools*, 1981, **12**, 205–210.

Shane, H. C., Lipschultz, R. W. and Shane, C. L. Facilitating the communicative interaction of nonspeaking persons in a residential setting. *Topics in Language Disorders*, 1982, **2**, 73–84.

Shere, B. and Kastenbaum, R. Mother-child interaction in cerebral palsy: Environmental and psychosocial obstacles to cognitive development. *Genetic Psychology Monographs*, 1966, **73**, 255–335.

Shipley, E., Gleitman, L. R. and Smith, C. A study in the acquisition of language: Free responses to commands. *Language*, 1969, **45**, 322–342.

Silverman, H., Kates, B. and McNaughton, S. The formative evaluation of the Ontario Crippled Children's Centre symbol communication program. In H. Silverman, S. McNaughton and B. Kates (Eds.), *Handbook of Blissymbolics*. Toronto: Ontario Crippled Children's Centre, 1978.

Sisson, L. A. and Barrett, R. P. An alternating treatment comparison of oral and total communication training with minimally verbal children. *Journal of Applied Behavior Analysis*, 1984, **17**, 559–566.

Siverts, B. E. *Sjekkliste for autister*. Oslo: Landsforeningen for Autister, 1982.

Skinner, B. F. *Verbal behavior*. New York: Appleton-Century-Crofts, 1957.

Skjelfjord, V. J. *Fonemlæring i skolen*. Oslo: Universitetsforlaget, 1976.

Smebye, H. K. Kommunikasjonsløse barn lærer å kommunisere på eget initiativ. *CP-Bladet*, 1984, **30**, 18–29.

Smebye, H. K. Kommunikasjonsinnlæring på barnets initiativ. *CP-Bladet*, 1985, **31**, 17–21.

Smebye, H. K. Strukturert overfortolkning. *CP-Bladet*, 1986, **32**, 19–26.

Smebye, H. K. Tom har lært å snakke. *CP-Bladet*, 1988, **34**, 5–9.

Smeets, P. M. and Striefel, S. Acquisition of sign reading by transfer of stimulus control in a retarded deaf girl. *Journal of Mental Deficiency Research*, 1976, **20**, 197–205.

Smith, A. K., Thurston, S., Light, J., Parnes, P. and O'Keele, B. The form and use of written communication produced by physically disabled individuals using microcomputers. *Augmentative and Alternative Communication*, 1989, **5**, 115–124.

Smith, C. *Communication link. A dictionary of signs.*

Middlesbrough: Beverly School for the Deaf, 1988.

Smith, L. and von Tetzchner, S. Communicative, sensorimotor, and language skills of young children with Down syndrome. *American Journal of Mental Deficiency*, 1986, **91**, 57–66.

Smith-Lewis, M. and Ford, A. A user's perspective on augmentative communication. *Augmentative and Alternative Communication*, 1987, **3**, 12–17.

Sommer, K. S., Whitman, T. L. and Keogh, D. A. Teaching severely retarded persons to sign interactively through the use of a behavioral script. *Research in Developmental Disabilities*, 1988, **9**, 291–304.

Sparrow, S. S., Balla, D. A. and Cicchetti, D. V. *Vineland Adaptive Behavior Scales. A revision of the Vineland Social Maturity Scale by Edgar A. Doll*. American Guidance Service, 1984.

Stokes, T. F., Baer, D. M. and Jackson, R. L. Programming the generalization of a greeting response in four retarded children. *Journal of Applied Behavior Analysis*, 1974, **7**, 599–610.

Sutton, A. C. Augmentative communication systems: The interaction process. Paper presented at the Annual Convention of the American Speech–Language–Hearing Association, Toronto, 1982.

Topper, S. T. Gesture language for a non-verbal severely retarded male. *Mental Retardation*, 1975, **13**, 30–31.

Trasher, K. and Bray, N. Effects of iconicity, taction, and training technique on the initial acquisition of manual signing by the mentally retarded. Paper presented at the Seventeenth Annual Gatinburg Conference on Research in Mental Retardation, Gatinburg, 1984.

Trefler, E. and Crislip, D. No aid, an Etran, a Minspeak: A comparison of efficiency and effectiveness during structured use. *Augmentative and Alternative Communication*, 1985, **1**, 151–155.

Trevinarus, J. and Tannock, R. A scanning computer access system for children with severe physical disabilities. *American Journal of Occupational Therapy*, 1987, **41**, 733–738.

Tronconi, A. Blissymbolics-based telecommunications. *Communication Outlook*, 1989, **11**, 8–11.

Undheim, J. O. *Håndbok til Wechsler Intelligence Scale for Children – Revised*. Oslo: Norsk Psykologforening, 1978.

Vanderheiden, D. B., Brown, W. P., MacKenzie, P., Reinen, S. and Scheibel, C. Symbol communication for the mentally handicapped. *Mental Retardation*, 1975, **13**, 34–37.

Vanderheiden, G. C. and Lloyd, L. L. Communication systems and their components. In S. W. Blackstone (Ed.), *Augmentative communication: An introduction*. Rockville, MD: American Speech and Hearing Association, 1986, pp. 49–161.

Villiers, J. G.D. and McNaughton, J. M. Teaching a symbol language to autistic children. *Journal of Consulting and Clinical Psychology*, 1974, **42**, 111–117.

van Osterom, J. and Devereux, K. *Learning with Rebus Glossary*. Black Hill, Cambs: EARO, The Resource Centre, 1985.

von Tetzchner, S. Facilitation of early speech development in a dysphatic child by use of signed Norwegian. *Scandinavian Journal of Psychology*, 1984a, **25**, 265–275.

von Tetzchner, S. Tegnspråksopplæring med psykotiske/autistiske barn: Teori, metode og en kasusbeskrivelse. *Tidsskrift for Norsk Psykologforening*, 1984b, **21**, 3–15.

von Tetzchner, S. Testprogrammer for barn med bevegelsesheming. Oslo: Sentralinstituttet for Cerebral Parese, 1987.

von Tetzchner, S. and Øien, I. Rett syndrom: Forløp og tiltak. Video. Oslo: Norsk forening for Rett syndrom, 1989.

Wagner, K.R. How much do children say in a day? *Journal of Child Language*, 1985, **12**, 475–487.

Walker, M. *Language programmes for use with the revised Makaton vocabulary*. Surrey: M. Walker, 1976.

Walker, M. and Ekeland, J. *The revised Makaton vocabulary, Norsk versjon (foreløpig utgave)*. Klæbu: Vernepleierhøgskolen i Sør-Trøndelag, 1985.

Walker, M., Parson, P., Cousins, S., Carpenter, B. and Park, K. *Symbols for Makaton*. Black Hill, Camps: EARO, The Resorce Centre, 1985.

Warren, S.F. and Kaiser, A.P. Incidental teaching: A critical review. *Journal of Speech and Hearing Disorders*, 1986, **51**, 291–299.

Watters, R.G. Wheeler, L.J. and Watters, W.E. The realtive efficiency of two orders for training autistic children in the expressive and receptive use of manual signs. *Journal of Communication Disorders*, 1981, 14, 273–285.

Webster, C.D., McPherson, L., Evans, M.A. and Kuchar, E. Communication with an autistic boy by gesture. *Journal of Autism and Childhood Schizophrenia*, 1973, 3, 337–346.

Weir, R.H. Some questions on the child's learning of phonology. In F. Smith and G.A. Miller (Eds.), *The genesis of language*. London: MIT Press, 1966, 153–168.

Weis, D.A. Cluttering. *Folia Phoniatrica*, 1967, 19, 233–263.

Wells, M.E. The effect of total communication training versus traditional speech training on word articulation in severely mentally retarded individuals. *Applied Research in Mental Retardation*, 1981, **2**, 323–333.

Wexler, K., Blau, A., Leslie, S. and Dore, J. Conversational interaction of nonspeaking cerebral palsied individuals and their speaking partners, with and without augmentative communication aids. Unpublished manuscript, West Haverstraw, Helen Hayes Hospital, 1983.

Wherry, J.N. and Edwards, R.P. A comparison of verbal, sign, and simultaneous systems for the acquisition of receptive language by an autistic boy. *Journal of Communication Disorders*, 1983, **16**, 201–216.

Wilbur, R.B. *American sign language and sign systems*. Baltimore, MD: University Park Press, 1979.

Wills, K.E. Manual communication for nonspeaking hearing children. *Journal of Pediatric Psychology*, 1981, **6**, 15–27.

Woodcock, R.W., Clark, C.R. and Davies, C.O. *Peabody Rebus Reading Program*. Circle Pines: American Guidance Service, 1969.

Yoder, D.E. and Kraat, A. Intervention issues in nonspeech communication. In J. Miller, D.E. Yoder and R.L. Schiefelbusch (Eds.), *Contemporary issues in language intervention*. Rockville, MD: American Speech and Hearing Association, 1983, pp. 27–51.

York, J., Nietupski, J. and Hamre-Nietupski, S. A decision-making process for using microswitches. *Journal of the Association for Persons with Severe Handicaps*, 1985, **10**, 214–223.

Yorkston, K.M., Honsinger, M.J., Dowden, P.A. and Marriner, N. Vocabulary selection: A case report. *Augmentative and Alternative Communication*, 1989, **5**, 101–109.

List of sign illustrations

Manual signs

Blissymbols

PIC signs

PCS